2-8-13

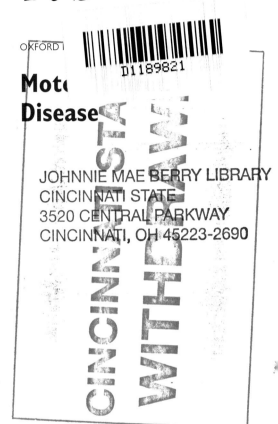

Published and forthcoming Oxford Care Manuals

Stroke Care: A Practical Manual
Rowan Harwood, Farhad Huwez, and Dawn Good

Multiple Sclerosis Care: A Practical Manual
John Zajicek, Jennifer Freeman, and Bernadette Porter (eds)

Dementia Care: A Practical Manual
Jonathan Waite, Rowan H. Harwood, Ian R. Morton, and
David J. Connelly

Headache: A Practical Manual
David Kernick and Peter J Goadsby (eds)

Diabetes Care: A Practical Manual
Rowan Hillson

Preventive Cardiology: A Practical Manual
Catriona Jennings, Alison Mead, Jennifer Jones, Annie Holden,
Susan Connolly, Kornelia Kotseva, and David Wood

Neuromuscular Disorders in the Adult: A Practical Manual
David Hilton-Jones, Jane Freebody, and Jane Stein

Oxford Care Manuals

Motor Neuron Disease

A Practical Manual

Kevin Talbot

Reader in Clinical Neurology and
Honorary Consultant Neurologist,
John Radcliffe Hospital, Oxford, UK

Martin R. Turner

Clinician Scientist and
Honorary Consultant Neurologist,
John Radcliffe Hospital, Oxford, UK

Rachael Marsden

Specialist Motor Neuron Disease Nurse,
John Radcliffe Hospital, Oxford, UK

Rachel Botell

Consultant in Neurorehabilitation,
Derriford Hospital, Plymouth, UK

OXFORD
UNIVERSITY PRESS

OXFORD
UNIVERSITY PRESS

Great Clarendon Street, Oxford OX2 6DP

Oxford University Press is a department of the University of Oxford.
It furthers the University's objective of excellence in research, scholarship,
and education by publishing worldwide in

Oxford New York

Auckland Cape Town Dar es Salaam Hong Kong Karachi
Kuala Lumpur Madrid Melbourne Mexico City Nairobi
New Delhi Shanghai Taipei Toronto

With offices in

Argentina Austria Brazil Chile Czech Republic France Greece
Guatemala Hungary Italy Japan Poland Portugal Singapore
South Korea Switzerland Thailand Turkey Ukraine Vietnam

Oxford is a registered trade mark of Oxford University Press
in the UK and in certain other countries

Published in the United States
by Oxford University Press Inc., New York

British Library Cataloguing in Publication Data
Data available

Library of Congress Cataloging in Publication Data
Data available

Typeset by Glyph International, Bangalore, India
Printed in Great Britain
on acid-free paper by
Ashford Colour Press Ltd, Gosport, Hampshire

ISBN 978–0–19–954736–4

10 9 8 7 6 5 4 3 2 1

Foreword

Not so long ago, in discussing motor neuron disease (MND) some standard textbooks of neurology elaborated the clinical features and differential diagnosis but had little or nothing positive to say about managing the condition. Indeed, the core concept of MND as a well-defined, rather homogeneous degenerative disorder of the upper and lower motor neurons remained largely unchallenged until two decades ago, despite some troubling dissonances – including the early recognition that cognition was not always normal, that pathological changes were not always restricted to the motor system, and that some individuals survived for many years after the predicted date of their demise. The identification of SOD1 gene mutations in 1993 heralded a new era. Not only has there been a rapid expansion of basic research, but the search for disease-modifying treatments has been intense, and not entirely fruitless. Most importantly, attitudes of neurologists and other health professionals to the care of people affected by MND have changed radically, reflecting a wholesale shift in the centre of gravity of neurology. This sociological change has moved in parallel with a thorough re-appraisal of the syndrome of MND. We face the uncomfortable recognition that there may be a dozen or more 'diseases' within the rubric of MND. For the clinician struggling to help patients with MND, this may be less of a problem than for the clinical scientist – after all, clinicians care for individuals, not categories. Nonetheless, any new text on MND – and particularly one in the Oxford Care Manuals series – should reconcile pragmatism, clinical common sense, and a clear didactic approach with our increasing recognition of complexity and uncertainty, while eschewing bias. As one would expect, the authors of this manual succeed admirably in surmounting these challenges. This addition to the series provides a practical, accessible, and authoritative summary of all aspects of current knowledge of MND from basic science through differential diagnosis and multi-disciplinary care. As such, I am sure it will be widely used and appreciated by students and teachers, novices and experts, health professionals and patients. I regard this manual as a landmark in the evolution of our struggle to improve the diagnosis and care of people with MND and related disorders, to find the means to halt the disease process, and ultimately to restore lost function.

Professor P. Nigel Leigh
King's MND Care and Research Centre
Department of Clinical Neuroscience
King's College London

Neuron or Neurone?

The term 'neuron' derives from the ancient Greek word, νευρον, meaning sinew or cord. It frequently appears, for example, in the muscular poetry of the Iliad of Homer. It was first coined in 1891 by Waldeyer (of the eponymous pharyngeal lymphoid ring) in the course of an article summarizing the findings of the great neuroscientist Ramon y Cajal. In his original German article he used the spelling 'neuron' as a direct transliteration of the Greek, without necessarily implying that he was coining a German word. Despite this, the French version of the word is *neurone*. In English, the addition of the 'e' appears to be on the basis that original ancient Greek pronunciation would have been with a long 'o' and so, to make phonological sense in English, an 'e' is required. However, the *Oxford English Dictionary* gives precedence to *neuron*, relegating *neurone* to the status of a variant.

Preface

The volume of published literature on the subject of motor neuron disease is increasing exponentially. Despite this, the rate of progress in developing effective treatments has been frustratingly slow. This book is not a synthesis of current clinical and scientific research into MND but rather a practical manual for those caring for patients living with the disease. However, in the modern era, patients with complex and intractable disease expect their physician to be knowledgeable about basic research. We have therefore provided some background information on the science underpinning MND and its variants. The focus of the remainder of the book is on the care of patients living with motor neuron disease, who rely on the skills and experience of a specialist multidisciplinary team to maintain their well-being in the face of one of the most challenging diseases in medicine.

Although a number of investigative aids are available (imaging, neurophysiology) MND remains a clinical diagnosis which can be reached using the same clinical tools available to neurologists in the 19th century. Understanding the individual patient phenotype is the key to planning care for a journey with the disease which, in the vast majority of cases, ends in death. With this in mind, we place great emphasis on understanding the clinical heterogeneity of motor neuron disease.

The management of MND is gradually becoming more 'evidence-based', but there are numerous areas where answers have to be synthesized from clinical experience and expert opinion. Although the information in this book is based on experience of managing approximately 500 patients with MND, such expertise as we offer here is, by its very nature, 'work in progress'.

Kevin Talbot
Martin R. Turner
Rachael Marsden
Rachel Botell

Oxford, UK
April 2009

Contents

Abbreviations

AAC	Augmentative and alternative communication aids
ADRT	Advance decision to refuse treatment
AFO	Ankle-foot orthosis
ALS	Amyotrophic lateral sclerosis
ALSFRS	ALS Functional Rating Scale
AR	Androgen receptor
bd	Twice daily
BDNF	Brain-derived neurotrophic factor
CIDP	Chronic inflammatory demyelinating polyneuropathy
CMAP	Compound muscle action potential
CNS	Central nervous system
CNTF	Ciliary neurotrophic factor
CPAP	Continuous positive airway pressure
CPK	Creatine phosphokinase
CST	Corticospinal tract
DLA	Disability Living Allowance
DTI	Diffusion tensor imaging
EHIC	European Health Insurance Card
EMG	Electromyography
ENU	Ethyl-N-nitrosourea
FA	Fractional anisotropy
fALS	Familial ALS
FBC	Full blood count
FOSMN	Facial onset sensory motor neuropathy
FTD	Frontotemporal dementia
FUS	Fused in sarcoma
GARS	Glycyl t-RNA synthetase
GDNF	Glial-derived neurotrophic factor
HAART	Highly active antiretroviral therapy
HRMC	Higher Rate Mobility Component
HSP	Hereditary spastic paraparesis
ICF	International Classification of Function
ICIDH	International Classification of Impairments, Disabilities, and Handicaps
IGF-1	Insulin-like growth factor
IM	Intramuscular
LFT	Liver function test
LPA	Lasting power of attorney
MAS	Mobile arm support

MAVIS	Mobility Advice & Vehicle Information Service
MDT	Multidisciplinary team
MMN	Multifocal motor neuropathy
MMT	Manual muscle testing
MND	Motor neuron disease
MRI	Magnetic resonance imaging
mtDNA	Mitochondrial DNA
MUNE	Motor unit number estimation
MVIC	Maximum voluntary isometric contraction
NCS	Nerve conduction studies
NGT	Nasogastric tube
NIV	Non-invasive ventilation
NMJ	Neuromuscular junction
NSAID	Non-steroidal anti-inflammatory drug
od	Once daily
OT	Occupational therapist
PBP	Progressive bulbar palsy
PE	Pulmonary embolism
PEG	Percutaneous endoscopic gastrostomy
PEJ	Percutaneous endoscopic jejunostomy
PLS	Primary lateral sclerosis
PMA	Progressive muscular atrophy
PPMA	Post-polio muscular atrophy
RIG	Radiologically inserted gastrostomy
qds	Four times daily
QoL	Quality of life
SACD	Sub-acute combined degeneration
sALS	Sporadic ALS
SBMA	Spinal and bulbar muscular atrophy
SMA	Spinal muscular atrophy
SNP	Sniff-nasal pressure
SOD	Superoxide dismutase
SSEP	Somatosensory evoked potentials
TDP-43	TAR-DNA binding protein
tds	Three times daily
TfL	Transport for London
TMS	Transcranial magnetic stimulation
TV	Tracheostomy ventilation
UBI	Ubiquitinated inclusion
ULN	Upper limit of normal
UMN	Upper motor neuron
WPMS	War Pensioner's Mobility Supplement

Background: understanding motor neuron disease

A note on terminology

It is unfortunate, and a source of much confusion, not least to patients, that different names are used when neurologists generally all agree that they are talking about the same clinical entity.

Motor neuron disease is used variously: (a) as an umbrella term for any disease in which motor neurons are the principal cell involved; (b) to describe conditions (e.g. ALS, PLS, PMA) falling within a recognised clinical spectrum of malignant neurodegenerative disorder with characteristic pathology; (c) as synonymous with amyotrophic lateral sclerosis, the most common form of degenerative disease of the motor neuron.

Amyotrophic lateral sclerosis, in its precise clinicopathological definition, refers to the form of motor neuron disease in which there is clear evidence of combined upper motor neuron and lower motor neuron involvement. 'ALS' is sometimes used loosely as a catch-all for all forms of late-onset degenerative motor neuron disease.

In this book, we use the terms MND and ALS interchangeably when such usage, in our judgement, is not likely to lead to confusion in the reader.

Brief historical background

- 1820–1850: recognition of the distinction between neurogenic and myopathic causes of muscle wasting.
- 1824: Bell may have described one of the first cases of ALS.
- 1850: Aran describes 'progressive muscular atrophy'.
- 1853: Cruveilhier describes atrophy of anterior roots and suspected malfunction of the anterior horn cells in cases of weakness.
- 1869: Charcot describes cases of 'amyotrophic lateral sclerosis' (a term first used in 1874) based upon his clinico-pathological observations of patients in whom there was a combination of muscle weakness and wasting (amotrophy) with sclerosis of the lateral columns at post-mortem, indicating upper motor neuron damage. Charcot believed that the failure of the anterior horn cell was secondary to malfunction of the corticospinal tract.
- 1875: Erb describes 'spastic spinal paralysis', widely taken to be the first description of the disorder we now recognise as primary lateral sclerosis.
- 1880s: Sir William Gowers argues that the upper and lower motor neuron components of the disease develop independently.
- 1930s: Russell Brain, in his book 'Diseases of the Nervous System', uses the term 'motor neuron disease' for the first time.
- 1940s: recognition of Western Pacific 'ALS'.
- 1993: identification of the first gene in which mutations lead to familial ALS (SOD1).
- 2008: identification of TDP-43 as the 'signature molecule' in the molecular pathological diagnosis of MND/ALS.

The nature of MND: one disease or many?

The answer to this question may depend on what we mean by a 'disease'. There are a number of levels of definition:

- **Clinical:** in this sense, MND is defined as a progressive pure motor syndrome with combined upper and lower motor neuron involvement in multiple territories with progression to death within a period of a few years. On a purely operational level we could consider MND as one disease on the grounds that neurologists mostly agree on what they mean by the term. However, this does not exclude the possibility that MND is a clinical syndrome with multiple different underlying aetiologies and pathologies.

- **Pathological:** MND is a neurodegenerative disease in which the pathological hallmark is the presence of ubiquitinated inclusions which stain with antibodies to the cellular protein TDP-43. Although this definition generally has a good correlation with the clinical definition of ALS, the fact that there are undoubtedly cases with different pathology but which are clinically indistinguishable from those with TDP-43 pathology (e.g. familial ALS due to SOD1 mutations) means that the correlation is not absolute.

- **Aetiological:** MND is a degenerative disease with a specific set of susceptibility factors which are typically unmasked by ageing processes. From the fact that there are forms of ALS which are familial (fALS) and due to mutations in a single gene and other forms of ALS which are sporadic (sALS), it is self evident that there are different aetiologies for this disease. Once we have established all of the possible causes of MND in their extreme complexity we may replace classifications based on clinical or pathological features with one based on a primary set of causes. Given that there are likely to be convergent pathways to neurodegeneration it may still be the case that diseases with different causes are responsive to the same treatments. Conversely, clinical syndromes that look superficially similar may require tailored disease-modifying therapy based on aetiology.

So, in considering what is not MND, we have to be mindful that an all-encompassing definition of what *is* MND is practically impossible. The modern view of MND emerging from genetic and pathological studies is that we are dealing with a clinico-pathological syndrome with a number of aetiologies. Furthermore, there is a previously unrecognised degree of complexity behind the apparently consistent clinical syndrome. Many different forms of familial MND are now defined. Sporadic MND may be a complex and heterogeneous disease with a large number of low-level genetic effects combining with environmental triggers and age-dependent stochastic changes in the nervous system. Each patient may therefore develop their disease for rather individual reasons.

Epidemiology

Incidence and prevalence

It will be self evident that the patients attending a specialist MND clinic in a tertiary referral centre do not represent all cases of the disease in a specific geographical area, and may contain an excess of patients with an atypical clinical course. Therefore, reliable data about the incidence and prevalence of the disease can only be obtained from population registries with robust methods of case definition and ascertainment. Such studies have only been performed thus far in developed countries with a predominantly European genetic heritage. We know relatively little about the epidemiology of MND in most parts of the world, including the most populous regions (China, India, and Africa). Therefore, the epidemiological study of MND is at present incomplete and it is appropriate to remain open-minded about the relative contribution of environmental factors.

These reservations aside, good-quality population-based epidemiological studies performed to date have demonstrated:

- An apparently uniform geographical incidence of around 1–2/100,000 population per year. While there is some apparent variation, published epidemiological studies vary in quality and it is important to distinguish between differences in methodology and true differences in incidence.
- No evidence that the incidence is either increasing or decreasing over time. Since the risk of MND increases with age, incidence rates must be corrected for changes in ageing demographics in a population. Consideration must also be given to whether apparent increases in incidence reflect better access to specialist healthcare and more rigorous case definition.
- A prevalence of 4–6/100,000 (compared with 800/100,000 for Alzheimer's disease, 160/100,000 for Parkinson's disease).
- The proportion of familial cases in population studies varies between 5–10%, presumably reflecting founder mutations and migration effects.
- A consistent excess of males over females which diminishes with age, such that over the age of 70 the ratio approaches unity.
- No convincing examples of population clusters for typical MND, indicating that environmental factors are either very modest or highly complex and difficult to identify.
- The only established risk factors for MND are therefore: age, male gender, and a family history of the disease (see Chapter 6 for a discussion of the genetic contribution to MND causation).

Environmental factors

Numerous environmental factors have been proposed, usually based on preconceived notions of disease causation. Approaches such as case-control studies, which generally depend on collecting data from patients based on closed questioning, are subject to false positive results due to recall bias. In general, the modest associations that have been reported between the risk of developing MND and environmental factors have not been replicated in subsequent studies. Like genetic association studies (see Chapter 6, Genetics of sporadic MND), environmental association studies seem to indicate that MND is a complex disease without causal determinants which exert a strong effect. In addition to a lack of any geographical variation in distribution, the absence of a significant increased risk in spouses of affected individuals argues against a temporally proximate environmental trigger for the disease.

Amongst the environmental exposures which have been considered candidates, but for which the evidence is lacking or provisional, a number are mentioned below, not least because they are often asked about by patients:

- **Physical profile**: a number of clinic-based studies suggest that athleticism is associated with the risk of MND, while population-based studies have yielded conflicting or negative results. There is a suggestion of an excess of sufferers among former service personnel and competitive athletes. A study which seemed to show that professional footballers in Italy had an eightfold excess risk has received particular attention. If there is an effect of athleticism on the risk of MND it may be that a genetic profile which promotes physical prowess in youth may confer deleterious physiological characteristics in the ageing nervous system. There is no evidence that exercise is harmful to people with established disease.
- **Heavy metals**: a number of metals (lead, mercury, cadmium, thallium, etc.) are neurotoxic and therefore plausible biological candidates for neurodegenerative disease. Such theories tend to have popular lay appeal. The clinical syndromes caused by acute heavy-metal toxicity are not typical of MND and are often reversible. Exposure of experimental animals to heavy metals does not recapitulate the pathological features of MND. The question is therefore whether low-level exposure over prolonged periods could be a contributory factor in a complex neurodegenerative disease, and this is much more difficult to refute. There is no clear association between occupational exposure to heavy metals and MND. Removal of amalgam dental fillings is appealing to patients and promoted by unscrupulous dentists, but there is no evidence that it slows progression of the disease, and anecdotal evidence suggests that it is harmful and produces much larger exposure to mercury during the removal procedure.
- **Trauma:** physical injury, such as long bone fracture, has been reported as an association in some case-control studies but not confirmed in others. There is no association between boxing and MND. Given that mild to moderate trauma is part of most people's life history, apparent associations are very likely to be subject to recall bias. There are case reports of MND occurring after electrical injury, but no increased incidence in electrical workers overall.

Age of onset

Data from population studies from around the world consistently show that the incidence of MND rises with age (see Figure 1.1). Age of onset is one of the most powerful prognostic factors in MND, with younger-onset patients generally having a slower disease course. It is thought that such younger-onset patients probably have a higher genetic component to their disease (although rarely a single gene defect, see Chapter 6).

Studies of clinic databases show that about one third of patients are under the age of 50 at symptom onset. The average age at symptom onset is approximately 60 years (consistently ~2 years older in women about the mean), and appears to be rising as the population ages and there is more equitable access to specialist care. Population-based studies invariably have a higher proportion of older patients, confirming that clinic studies are biased towards younger patients (see Table 1.1).

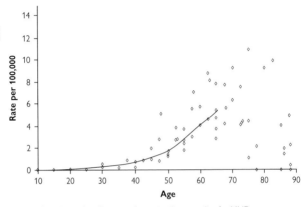

Fig. 1.1 Cumulative data from population incidence studies for MND (reproduced with permission from Hirtz et al. (2007) How common are the common neurologic disorders? *Neurol* 68; 326–337).

Table 1.1 The profile of age of onset in MND compared between a typical study based on a specialist clinic and a population-based study.

Clinic database (831 patients) (Havercamp et al., 1995)		Population study (517 patients) (Beghi et al., 2007)	
Age of onset	Percentage of MND population	Age of onset	Percentage of MND population
21–30	4%	–	–
31–40	10%	<45	9%
41–50	15%	45–55	13%
51–60	30%	55–64	28%
61–70	30%	65–74	33%
>70	11%	>75	17%

Survival

Survival is heterogeneous in MND, with a wide range around a mean of 3–4 years from symptom onset (range six months to 20 years). The median survival for typical ALS is 30 months from first symptoms and 20 months from diagnosis. The most consistent predictor of survival is the rate of progression of the disease in the first year. Rapid acceleration of progression or a 'plateau' phase once the initial rate is established are exceptional. Collectively, the prognosis of all forms of MND is shown in Figure 1.2 with data from the Scottish Motor Neuron Disease register:

• The cumulative probability of survival is 54% at 2 years from diagnosis.
• Survival did not improve over a 10 year period.

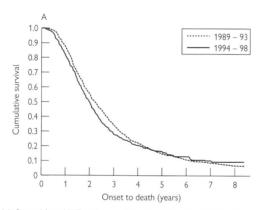

Fig. 1.2 Survival from MND in the population-based Scottish MND register (reproduced from Forbes *et al.* (2004) Unexpected decline in survival from amyotrophic lateral sclerosis/motor neurone disease. *J Neurol* 75; 1753–5, with permission from BMJ Publishing Group Ltd).

• The variation in natural history of specific syndromes within MND is covered in Chapter 3.
• See Chapter 12 for a discussion of prognosis in individual patients.

Neuropathology

The earliest descriptions of ALS, by Charcot and others, were made at the time when neuropathology was becoming an established discipline and the 'definition' of ALS has become inextricably linked with a series of pathological changes, or disease 'hallmarks'. It is important to appreciate that the neuropathological approach to understanding neurodegenerative disease has limitations as well as advantages:

• Neuropathology ('morbid neuroanatomy') is fundamentally descriptive rather than mechanistic. It does not follow that common phenomenology between brains of ALS patients necessarily represents a unified cause.

• Neuropathology is by necessity a cross-sectional approach to the study of disease with one observational time-point, remote from disease initiation

• The architecture of the nervous system, and the chemistry of tissue-staining methods lead to a preferential focus on changes in the cell body. Over 95% of the volume of a motor neuron is contained in the cell processes and the physiologically functional pole of any neuron is the synapse, neither of which can easily be visualised in conventional neuropathological analysis. The apparently simple demonstration of changes in neuronal number is fraught with methodological controversies.

• The tissue available at the end stage of a progressive neurological disease like ALS contains cells that have 'survived'. The cells that have been lost resulting in the death of the patient are in principle of more interest to the research investigator, if not to the diagnostic pathologist. However, in any sample of brain and spinal cord from an ALS patient it is likely that there will also be areas of the nervous system in which the disease process may be at an early stage.

Charcot appreciated in the 1870s that cells in the spinal cord of patients with ALS contained 'debris'. An important advance came in the 1980s when the specificity of intraneuronal inclusion bodies which stain for ubiquitin in ALS spinal cord and brain came to be recognised as a hallmark of the disease. Finally, in 2008 TAR-DNA binding protein (TDP-43) was identified as the major protein component of ubiquitinated inclusions which define a spectrum of 'TDP-43 proteinopathies', from lower motor neuron predominant ALS, through typical Charcot ALS, to frontotemporal dementia with or without motor neuron degeneration.

Inclusion bodies in **MND/ALS**

- Ubiquitinated inclusions (UBIs) are present in the spinal cord of 100% of patients with a clinical diagnosis of sporadic ALS. TDP-43 is the major protein constituent and, in cells with UBIs, it is displaced from its normal location in the nucleus. UBIs have a range of morphologies ranging from spherical to 'skein-like'.

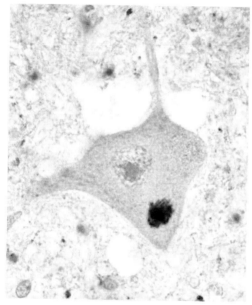

Fig. 1.3 Ubiquitinated cytoplasmic inclusion in ventral horn motor neuron from the spinal cord of a patient with typical ALS (courtesy of Dr Olaf Ansorge, Department of Neuropathology, John Radcliffe Hospital, Oxford).

- Bunina bodies: eosinophilic, paracrystalline, present in >85% of ALS cases; immunoreactive for the proteinase inhibitor cystatin C.
- Hyaline inclusions: these occur with a lower frequency than UBIs and are particularly present in familial SOD1 mutation cases (especially I113T and A4V); immunoreactive for neurofilaments.

Sporadic ALS

- **Motor cortex:** there are examples of patients with clear upper motor neuron signs in life and normal motor cortex at autopsy, and it has been difficult to establish any consistent correlation between clinical features and the loss of motor neurons in the motor cortex. Ubiquitinated inclusions are generally less common than in the spinal cord. However, several studies have demonstrated Bunina bodies in the motor cortex of patients with a clinical diagnosis of 'lower motor neuron disease'/progressive muscular atrophy in life, providing strong support for the inclusion of PMA in the spectrum of ALS/MND. Variable degrees of astrocytic gliosis and microglial activation are also found in the motor cortex.
- **Corticospinal tract (CST):** loss of axons, myelin pallor and gliosis are found in the CST in ALS, including in cases classified in life as having a pure lower motor neuron form of the disease.
- **Brainstem:** in keeping with the clinical observation of sparing of the extraocular muscles, the motor nuclei of cranial nerves III, IV and VI are not affected.
- **Spinal cord:** typically there is a 50% loss of spinal motor neurons. Surviving cells show atrophy or abnormal staining. Whether there is clear evidence of apoptosis is still controversial.
- **Peripheral nerve:** the ventral roots are severely atrophic. The dorsal root ganglia frequently show detectable cell loss. There are reduced numbers of axons in the nerve trunk, but demyelination is a secondary feature.
- **Neuromuscular junction and muscle:** in the SOD1 mouse model of familial ALS neuromuscular junction disruption precedes degeneration of the cell body in the spinal cord, but NMJs have not been extensively studied in humans with ALS. Muscle shows evidence of denervation and re-innervation (fibre-type grouping).
- **Extramotor areas of the CNS:** although typical ALS patients have a disorder entirely restricted to the motor system in terms of clinical findings, on pathological grounds ALS is a diffuse multisystem neurodegenerative process. Patients who have survived beyond their 'natural' disease course because of invasive artificial ventilation show very extensive neurodegeneration in widespread regions of the CNS. The areas most frequently involved include the spinocerebellar tract, ascending dorsal column sensory pathways and thalamus, and the substantia nigra. The dentate gyrus of the hippocampal formation and the frontal and temporal neocortex show UBIs in 30% of ALS patients, who in life typically have subtle sub-clinical evidence of extramotor involvement in the form of mild dysexecutive problems (see Chapter 3).

Familial ALS

Information on the pathology of fALS is sparse and mostly limited to SOD1, where there is a suggestion that hyaline conglomerate inclusions are more common than in sporadic ALS. Crucially, TDP-43 is absent in SOD1 cases, lending support to the idea that this condition is pathologically distinct from sALS and other forms of fALS.

Animal models of motor neuron disease

There is no known, naturally occurring, spontaneous, age-dependent neurodegenerative disease with the pathological appearance of ALS in animals. Such animal models as exist therefore have an indirect relationship to ALS, not least because of the unique properties of the human corticospinal tract.

- The identification of genetic defects leading to motor neuron degeneration that have arisen spontaneously in in-bred strains of laboratory mice has produced important insights into motor neuron function but the relevance for ALS is not clear. Examples include the *progressive motor neuronopathy* mouse (mutations in the tubulin-specific chaperone, Tbce) and the *wobbler* mouse (mutations in the vesicle sorting protein, VPS54)
- Mouse mutants from programs of systematic mutagenesis with genotoxins such as ENU can show motor neuron phenotypes, e.g. the *loa* mouse with mutations in dynein.
- Models in dogs (e.g. canine spinal muscular atrophy due to mutations in FVT1) have so far been more like non-ALS motor neuron disorders. Canine degenerative myelopathy (DM) is due to a E40K mutation in the SOD1 gene. The disease appears to be recessive and histopathologically distinct from sporadic ALS.
- Horses can develop spontaneous motor neuron disease which appears to be due, at least in part, to vitamin E deficiency.

Transgenic mouse models

The first mice carrying transgenic copies of mutant forms of the human SOD1 gene were created in 1995. The most commonly used model (SOD1 G93A) develops weakness at about 2.5 months post-natally and dies by 4–4.5 months.

- The mice contain many (>20) copies of the mutant gene and produce high levels of mutant protein.
- The disease is fully penetrant and has a stereotyped course.
- Numerous drugs appear to confer survival benefit, typically a few weeks.
- None of these agents has translated into an effective therapy in human ALS trials.
- As with familial ALS cases with SOD1 mutations, SOD1 transgenic mice do not demonstrate TDP-43 pathology.
- Transgenic mouse models expressing mutant TDP-43 have been produced and may provide new insights into the pathogenesis of motor neuron death.

Summary of proposed pathological mechanisms in ALS

Almost all knowledge about the pathophysiology of motor neuron degeneration in ALS comes either from inferences drawn from cellular changes post-mortem or from the SOD1 transgenic mouse model. Current concepts of motor neuron 'selective vulnerability' fail to consider the cell within the context of the motor system as a whole. The following pathways have been proposed to be important in ALS, and there are shared themes between ALS and other neurodegenerative diseases:

- Protein misfolding: the presence of intraneuronal aggregates positive for ubiquitin implies that misfolded protein accumulates in degenerating motor neurons. As with other neurodegenerative diseases there is an ongoing argument as to whether aggregates are toxic (e.g. by inhibiting proteosome or chaperone function), protective (through the removal of toxic products), or incidental (i.e. reflect normal disposal of misfolded protein).
- Mitochondrial abnormalities are an early feature of pathology in the SOD1 mouse models. Mutant SOD1 has been shown to localise to the inner mitochondrial membrane. Mitochondria are a critical mediator of programmed cell death. Other human diseases associated with mitochondrial dysfunction, however, involve multiple physiological systems and are not confined to the nervous system.
- Axonal transport: the accumulation of neurofilaments, the major protein in axons, is a cardinal feature of human ALS and mouse models. Motor neurons are the longest cells in the body and axonal transport is critical. A number of inherited motor disorders are due to mutations in proteins relevant to axonal function (e.g. KIF1b in Charcot-Marie-Tooth Disease Type 2a).
- Excitotoxicity: glutamate is the main excitatory neurotransmitter in the CNS but is toxic to neurons. Astrocytes have membrane transporters for glutamate uptake. Motor neurons are more sensitive to glutamate-mediated excitotoxicity because of post-transcriptional editing of the GluR2 receptor which makes the cell more sensitive to Ca^{2+}. There is also evidence of failure of upstream control of excitatory neurons by inhibitory interneurons.
- Apoptosis: there is evidence that motor neurons have a specific pathway to programmed cell death through the fas-receptor and nitric oxide.
- Oxidative stress: motor neurons are large, highly energetic cells. Post-mortem studies reveal that reactive oxygen species and oxidative damage of protein are more abundant in ALS tissue. The possible 'gain of function' mechanism for SOD1 cellular toxicity may involve abnormal redox chemistry. Antioxidants, however, have not proved to be therapeutically effective in clinical trials.
- Contribution of other cell types: evidence from mouse models in which specific subtypes of cells have expressed SOD1 mutants indicates that microglia make a significant contribution to ALS pathogenesis.

References and further reading

Beghi E, Millul A, Micheli A, Vitelli E, Logroscino G for the SLALOM Group (2007). Incidence of ALS in Lombardy, Italy. *Neurology*, 68, 141–145.

Bruijn LI, Miller TM, Cleveland DW (2004). Unraveling the mechanisms involved in motor neuron degeneration in ALS. *Annu Rev Neurosci*, 27, 723–49.

Forbes RB, Colville S, Cran GW, Swingler RJ (2004). Unexpected decline in survival from amyotrophic lateral sclerosis/motor neurone disease. *J Neurol Neurosurg Psychiatry*, 75, 1753–1755.

Haverkamp LJ, Appel V, Appel SH (1995). Natural history of amyotrophic lateral sclerosis in a database population. Validation of a scoring system and a model for survival prediction. *Brain*, 118, 707–19.

Hirtz D, Thurman DJ, Gwinn-Hardy K, Mohamed M, Chaudhuri AR, Zalutsky R (2007). How common are the 'common' neurologic disorders? *Neurology*, 68, 326–337.

Diagnosis: is it motor neuron disease?

Diagnostic delay

Evidence suggests that neurologists are good at diagnosing MND, but that non-specialists may make diagnostic errors. Despite the reliability of neurological diagnosis, a number of factors lead to diagnostic delay:

- The onset of the disease is insidious and subtle, usually over months.
- Patients will often rationalise weakness as due to a 'trapped nerve' or some other reversible condition and delay visiting a primary care doctor.
- General practitioners are likely to be relatively unfamiliar with neurological disease and to fail to elicit physical signs early in the illness.
- There may be delays in accessing a specialist neurological opinion in some areas.
- The neurologist will initiate a series of investigations to exclude other disorders, which may take time.
- MND is a grave diagnosis to offer a patient and, even when there may be no other realistic considerations, neurologists may delay conveying the diagnosis to patients until the physical signs are consistent with criteria-based diagnostic schemes.
- Depending on cultural factors, it may be considered compassionate to delay conveying the diagnosis in a situation where there are no significant disease modifying treatments.

These factors explain why the average diagnostic delay for MND is about 1 year. Diagnostic delay is one of the most robust surrogate markers of survival identified to date. The relationship is inverse: rapidly progressing cases tend to present sooner to tertiary services and are associated with a worse survival.

Potential consequences of diagnostic delay

- The therapeutic window for disease-modifying treatments may be missed and clinical trials occur too late, increasing the possibility of missing a true treatment effect.
- Delayed care planning and promotion of crisis management.
- Distress and frustration for the patient, loss of confidence in medical professionals, and unnecessary investigations.
- Interventions for which there is evidence of benefit such as PEG (see Chapter 10) and NIV (see Chapter 9) may be delayed.

Clinical diagnosis of motor neuron disease

The presentation and natural history of different clinical patterns of MND is described in Chapter 3, but in all cases the following important principles must be observed (see also Box 2.1):

- Could the clinical symptoms and signs be explained by a structural lesion at one anatomical site? If yes, then imaging is mandatory.
- Is there a pure motor syndrome? If not, then other diagnoses must be considered.
- Is there progression? If not, the diagnosis of MND cannot be made
- Is there weakness? If not, the diagnosis of MND must be questioned and should probably remain provisional
- Have other disorders which could mimic MND been considered and excluded?
- MND is a *clinical* diagnosis. Paraclinical investigations such as neurophysiology and imaging have a vital role in excluding ALS mimics (see Investigation of suspected motor neuron disease, p. 22) but must be interpreted in the context of the clinical findings.

Site of first symptoms

How symptom onset (the clinical horizon) relates to pathological onset is not certain, but neurophysiological studies in pre-symptomatic carriers of SOD1 mutations suggests an acute decline in motor unit number approximately 6–9 months prior to clinically manifest disease. 98% of patients with MND can clearly identify the region of the body where they first noticed their symptoms. Although this is usually referred to as the 'site of onset', it remains an open question whether the pathological process in MND is truly focal in onset. At diagnosis the majority of patients will show evidence on examination of more diffuse involvement. Such evidence as exists indicates that in classical ALS upper and lower motor neuron pathways may be affected synchronously. The approximate distribution of site of onset is:

- Weakness of the upper limb ('spinal onset')   35%
- Weakness of the lower limb ('spinal onset')   30%
- Difficulty in speaking and swallowing ('bulbar onset')   30%
- Axial weakness (difficulty with erect posture or 'dropped head')   3%
- Respiratory symptoms ('respiratory onset')   <2%

The 'dropped head' (due to neck weakness) should raise suspicions of ALS, although myasthenia gravis and myopathy are other considerations.

Spread

One of the most characteristic clinical features of MND is the fact that patients will report worsening at each clinic visit. Given this progression the question arises whether MND spreads in a random or an orderly pattern. This seemingly simple question has profound significance for understanding the pathophysiology of the disease. If the disease spreads in an anatomically defined way, then the identification of the mechanism of this spread would have major implications for development of therapies to arrest the disease process. If the spread appears to be random, then this suggests either a diffuse degenerative disease or a multifocal one. In either case it is difficult to conceive of a mechanism whereby a catastrophic failure of groups of neurons in different locations would occur essentially synchronously without the action of some 'circulating' factor which might be detectable in the blood or CSF. Natural history studies have demonstrated that neurological dysfunction in one limb will, as described by the patient, spread to the contralateral limb in the same region (i.e. arm to arm, leg to leg) or to the ipsilateral limb in an adjacent region (e.g. R arm to R leg). Underlying this observation is a complex mixture of upper and lower motor neuron signs which make it difficult to draw firm conclusions about the anatomical basis of this apparently contiguous spread.

Box 2.1 'Red flags' in MND diagnosis

- Symptoms and signs explainable by a lesion at one anatomical site.
- Lack of progression, or major fluctuations in function.
- Prominent sensory symptoms and objective sensory signs.
- Prominent pain.
- Absence of weakness.
- Symmetry.
- Weakness without wasting.

Investigation of suspected motor neuron disease

The question of how intensively to investigate a suspected case of MND is the source of much anxiety. Despite the high level of diagnostic accuracy among neurologists and the unmistakable clinical features of typical 'Charcot ALS', diagnosis is still often delayed in some patients while the neurologist seeks certainty. It is not possible to be prescriptive herein about when to stop investigating, but simply to offer some general guidelines (see Boxes 2.2, 2.3). Neurology is practiced in a wide variety of settings which influence the prior probability of a particular diagnosis. Early presentations of what ultimately turns out to be MND can be subtle, and a period of further clinical observation, and repeated tests, can be appropriate before committing to a firm diagnosis. The degree of investigation of a suspected case of MND may be dictated by a number of non-clinical factors:

- In tertiary referral specialist MND clinics, patients arrive having been filtered by one or more neurological specialists, and with the passage of time the clinical features have matured. This makes the diagnosis considerably easier, and further investigation is often unnecessary.
- Specialist centres may have a research program which includes non-routine investigation or may simply seek to be definitive, so that all concerned can draw a line under the diagnostic phase and concentrate on management.
- Patients are increasingly well informed and may drive further investigation. While this may be challenging for clinicians, a pragmatic approach is required. If sensitive and open discussion about how the diagnosis is achieved does not produce resolution, it may occasionally be very difficult to engage patients in management without further investigation.

Imaging

- In modern neurological practice it would be exceptional to make a diagnosis of MND without performing imaging, usually MRI, with the aim of excluding other pathologies which can mimic the disease. Exceptions might include patients with clear upper and lower motor neuron signs above and below the neck at presentation and typical EMG findings, or patients who are unable to tolerate MRI because of orthopnoea.
- A minority (<40%) of patients with typical clinical MND have T2 hyperintensity in the corticospinal tract on MRI. The significance of this is unknown but it is not an indication of some other disease process (see Figure 2.1). It is also non-specific and can occur in other disorders.
- Patients with bulbar onset and tongue wasting are less likely to have an alternative diagnosis. In this case, if there are no atypical features, and especially if there are other features supportive of MND, MRI is usually performed, but clinical discretion can apply. However, spastic dysarthria without evidence of tongue wasting has a significant differential diagnosis and brain imaging is mandatory.

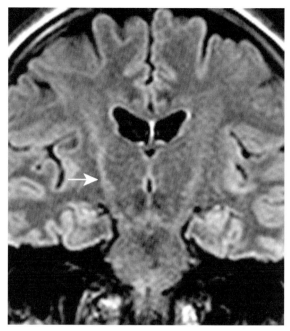

Fig. 2.1 T2-weighted coronal MRI scan in a young patient with rapidly progressive ALS demonstrating hyperintensity in the corticospinal tracts (courtesy of Dr Pieter Pretorius, Department of Neuroradiology, John Radcliffe Hospital, Oxford).

- Cervical spinal pathology can be particularly varied in its manifestations. The investigation of patients with limb-onset weakness and wasting, with or without upper motor neuron signs, should always include an MRI of the spine. If this is normal, selected patients, especially those with a predominantly upper motor neuron picture with modest or questionable muscle wasting, require brain imaging.
- Spinal imaging is normal in MND, but degenerative disease is very common in the target age group and must be interpreted in the light of the clinical findings if unnecessary surgery is to be avoided.
- Conventional structural MRI cannot detect change in functional anatomical pathways and is therefore not suitable as a marker of disease progression. Diffusion MRI techniques such as tractography are under investigation as a potential biomarker of disease progression (see Imaging, Chapter 5).

Neurophysiology

The motor unit is the collective term for one anterior horn cell, its axon, and the muscle fibres it innervates. It is believed that at least 30% of motor units must be lost before there is clinically evident weakness and wasting. This reflects the capacity for surviving motor units to collaterally innervate adjacent muscle fibres.

The neurophysiological hallmarks of classical ALS are:

- normal motor nerve and sensory nerve conduction
- fibrillation and fasciculation potentials
- reduced motor unit potentials and increased amplitude and duration of remaining motor units.

It would be difficult for most neurologists to imagine making a diagnosis of MND without access to clinical neurophysiology. In some cases it can be vital in confirming a clinical suspicion of MND. Even more importantly, in rare situations neurophysiology can provide concrete evidence of another disorder which mimics MND, such as conduction block neuropathy. However, it is true that in many typical cases of MND an abnormal EMG merely confirms what is clinically obvious and an undue reliance on EMG 'criteria' can interfere with the important matter of coming to a clinical diagnosis.

- EMG is a sampling technique and therefore the probability of detecting an abnormality is a function of the extent of denervation and the amount of time devoted to the test. Therefore, it should not be surprising if occasional patients with clinically probable MND appear to have little or no evidence of denervation on EMG.
- EMG is of particular value in demonstrating more widespread evidence of denervation in patients with clinical symptoms and signs restricted to one limb. Similarly it may provide evidence of denervation of the tongue, which is helpful in confirming widespread degeneration in cases where the differential diagnosis is degenerative spinal cord disease.
- In patients with fasciculations only, EMG can distinguish benign from MND-type fasciculations with a reasonable degree of certainty. However, the diagnosis of benign fasciculations can frequently be made confidently without resorting to neurophysiology.
- Patients with progressive bulbar palsy, by which is meant an upper motor neuron predominant disorder initially isolated to speech and swallowing, may have a normal EMG. In this context the diagnosis (and planning of PEG feeding) should be made on clinical grounds.
- It is claimed that serial EMG can provide prognostic information which can help management planning. However, it has not clearly been established that this is better than clinical rating scales, measures of respiratory function, or expert clinical opinion. In most clinical settings, neurophysiology is a scarce resource and it is not practical (or necessarily acceptable to the patient) to perform repeated testing.
- EMG techniques such as motor unit number estimation (MUNE) continue to be an important research tool illuminating the basic pathophysiology of MND and may have a role as a potential biomarker (see Neurophysiology, Chapter 5).

- The upper motor neuron can be explored experimentally using transcranial magnetic stimulation (TMS). This has demonstrated that MND patients have a failure of cortical inhibition.

Lumbar puncture

Examination of the cerebrospinal fluid in suspected MND has a potential role as a biomarker but is only appropriate for selected patients in normal clinical practice.

- Routinely available CSF measures (cell count, protein, and glucose) are normal in MND.
- In any situation where the clinical picture is atypical it would be reasonable to perform an examination of the CSF.
- A raised CSF protein can be helpful in possible cases of pure motor CIDP.
- Very rarely, multiple sclerosis can produce focal wasting in association with corticospinal tract signs, so a relapsing and remitting course in an apparent case of spinal-onset MND should prompt a test for oligoclonal bands.
- Any features raising the suggestion of paraneoplastic neurological disease should be investigated with a lumbar puncture (including oligoclonal bands).

Box 2.2 Essential investigations in suspected MND

- Full blood count and ESR.
- Full biochemical profile including calcium.
- Creatine kinase (non-sensitive: usually mildly elevated or normal; >1000 iu/L is very unusual in MND).
- Thyroid function.
- Serum electrophoresis.
- Nerve conduction studies and EMG.
- MRI spine/brain as indicated by clinical signs.

Box 2.3 Additional investigations in selected cases

- B12 and methylmalonic acid (latter for functional B12 deficiency).
- Anti-neuronal antibodies for paraneoplastic disease.
- Anti-acetylcholine-receptor antibodies.
- HIV serological tests.
- Lyme serology.
- Lumbar puncture.
- Muscle biopsy.

El Escorial diagnostic criteria

Motor neuron disease is a clinical diagnosis in which special investigations have a role in confirming the diagnosis and excluding potential mimic conditions. The ideal diagnostic scheme should lead to the inclusion of all cases of a disease and exclusion of all cases of mimic syndromes. The El Escorial criteria (1994) and a subsequent revision (2000) are accepted as the standard way to include and exclude patients from therapeutic trials and other research studies (www.wfnals.org). However, it is generally acknowledged that the criteria are too stringent for clinical practice and do not improve the diagnostic accuracy of an experienced neurologist. Rigid dependence on these criteria for clinical diagnosis is likely to contribute to diagnostic delay. The four 'regions' referred to in the El Escorial criteria are bulbar, cervical, thoracic, and lumbosacral.

Box 2.4 El Escorial diagnostic criteria

The diagnosis of Amyotrophic Lateral Sclerosis (ALS) requires:

A – the presence of:
(A:1) evidence of lower motor neuron (LMN) degeneration
by clinical, electrophysiological, or neuropathologic examination, and
(A:2) evidence of upper motor neuron (UMN) degeneration
by clinical examination, and
(A:3) progressive spread of symptoms or signs within a region or to other regions, as determined by history or examination,

together with:

B – the absence of:
(B:1) electrophysiological and pathological evidence of other disease processes that might explain the signs of LMN and/or UMN degeneration, and
(B:2) neuroimaging evidence of other disease processes that might explain the observed clinical and electrophysiological signs.

Hierarchy of diagnosis under the El-Escorial scheme

Definite ALS
- UMN signs and LMN signs in three regions (bulbar, arm, leg).

Probable ALS
- UMN signs and LMN signs in two regions with at least some UMN signs rostral to LMN signs.

Probable ALS-Laboratory supported
- UMN signs in one or more regions and LMN involvement defined by EMG in at least two regions.

Possible ALS
- UMN signs and LMN signs in one region.
- UMN signs in two or more regions.
- UMN signs and LMN signs in two regions with no UMN signs rostral to LMN signs.

Note that:
- There is no category which allows for pure LMN disease, despite evidence that progressive muscular atrophy (PMA) is pathologically within the ALS spectrum (see Chapter 1).
- Significant numbers of patients do not fulfil the criteria at a stage when they would be ideal candidates for clinical trials.
- Terms such as 'probable' and 'possible' lead to frustration in patients who, very reasonably, look to their physicians for diagnostic clarity.

MND mimics

An MND mimic is any condition which may present with similar clinical features and be misdiagnosed as MND. The list of conditions which can apparently mimic MND is very long, though many of these are the subjects of small series or individual case reports. Clinic populations are biased by referral patterns and the research interests of individual clinicians, and may give an incorrect estimate of the true incidence of mis-diagnosis.

- Population-based surveys have indicated that over 8% of patients who are diagnosed with MND ultimately turn out to have another condition. (See Table 2.1, taken from Logroscino *et al.* 2008)
- A few conditions account for the majority of these misdiagnoses: compressive myelopathy, other neurodegenerative syndromes, inflammatory neuropathies, and other motor neuron disorders.
- The importance of identifying MND mimics relates mostly to the early phase of disease in which the concern is to identify treatable conditions. True cases of MND almost always declare themselves with time.

Table 2.1 Revised diagnoses of patients with amyotrophic lateral sclerosis mimic syndromes referred to two population based registries

Revised diagnosis	No of patients
Scottish Registry (years 1989–1992: n=552 patients)	
Cervical spondylotic myeloradiculopathy	10
'MND plus' syndromes	7
Cerebrovascular disease	5
Radiculopathy of unknown cause	4
Probable multiple sclerosis	4
Multiple system atrophy	4
Peripheral neuropathy of unknown cause	4
Multifocal motor neuropathy	2
Other	9
Uncertain	4
Total	53

Table 2.1 Revised diagnoses of patients with amyotrophic lateral sclerosis mimic syndromes referred to two population based registries (*continued*)

Revised diagnosis	No. of patients
Irish Registry (years 1993–1997; n=437 patients)	
Multifocal motor neuropathy	7
Kennedy disease	4
Motor neuropathy	3
Non-compressive myelopathy	21
Spinomuscular atrophy	2
Other	6
Uncertain	8
Total	32

Reproduced from Logroscino G et al. (2008). Descriptive epidemiology of amyotrophic lateral sclerosis: new evidence and unresolved issues. J Neurol Neurosurg Psychiatry, 79; 6–11, with permission of BMJ Publishing Group Ltd.

MND-like disorders lacking TDP-43 pathology

The following are conditions which may be clinically indistinguishable from the ALS spectrum, even until death, but in which the pathology is distinct, implying that the pathogenesis is different. Since there are no systematic post-mortem studies of populations of patients with MND we have no real way of identifying the true incidence of such 'phenocopies', however it is likely to be low.

- *Motor neuron disease with basophilic inclusions* has been described mostly in juvenile or young adult patients (almost all women) with rapidly progressive and symmetrical lower motor neuron degeneration. Histologically, the inclusions contain RNA and associated proteins. This is a very rare condition which currently can only be diagnosed *post mortem*. Originally described in young Japanese women, it should be considered in any young patient.
- *The ALS-Parkinsonian-Dementia complex* occurs on the Pacific Island of Guam and a similar disorder occurs in the Kii Peninsula of Japan and in a region of Papua New Guinea. Collectively these disorders have been referred to as 'Western Pacific ALS'. On Guam, at least, this seems to be an environmentally determined neurodegenerative disorder which is now declining in incidence. The pathology is distinct from ALS and is dominated by tau-positive neurofibrillary tangles. Despite intense research the relative contribution of environmental factors and a genetically susceptible population remains obscure. The cycad neurotoxicity hypothesis has now largely been refuted.

- *Familial ALS due to mutations in SOD1*, more controversially, could now be considered to be a disease with a different pathology which can mimic sporadic ALS and all other forms of fALS in which TDP-43 staining is a pathological hallmark.

Cervical spondylotic myeloradiculopathy

- One of the commonest ALS mimics.
- Most frequent cause of spastic paraparesis.
- Dual pathology is a diagnostic problem: many patients in the MND age-group have degenerative spine disease. About 4% have undergone inappropriate spinal surgery before MND is recognized.
- Clinical clue: UMN signs caudal to LMN signs in cervical spine disease.
- L'hermitte's sign (electric shock-like lancinations on neck flexion) is suggestive.
- Presentation is variable, and often spares sphincters until very late in the course.
- Stiff legs and loss of manual dexterity are the commonest presentation.
- Typical course: initial progressive phase then plateau.
- Pain is usually a feature.
- 80% have some sensory complaints but pure motor presentations do occur, making the differentiation from ALS problematic.

Other causes of myelopathy

These are unlikely to be confused with MND but should be considered in any patients with a spastic paraparesis, with or without sensory disturbance:

- Sub-acute combined degeneration (SACD): measure B12; if normal, and strong clinical suspicion, measure methylmalonic acid and homocysteine levels to exclude a functional deficiency due to cellular transport failure mechanisms.
- Copper deficiency myelopathy has an SACD-like presentation with anaemia. It is usually a consequence of chronic malabsorption, but high-dose oral zinc supplements can also precipitate it through competitive transport.
- Primary progressive multiple sclerosis (MRI brain and cord, evoked potential studies, and LP including oligoclonal bands may be indicated).
- Adrenomyeloneuropathy (measure very long chain fatty acid levels).

Diseases mimicking bulbar MND

As with any patient presenting with MND, the key question is whether the signs and symptoms can be explained by structural disease at one anatomical site. A large number of potential mimics of bulbar MND have been described but only rarely will these be confused with MND. Important things to consider include:

- Intrinsic lesions of the brainstem such as aneurysms, vascular disease, and demyelination. These will almost always cause signs that are inconsistent with MND such as dysconjugate gaze or trigeminal sensory loss.
- Myasthenia gravis (MG) – variation in symptoms, with fatiguability, is the hallmark of MG; extraocular muscles are very frequently involved.

- Cerebrovascular disease can cause spastic dysarthria and emotionality but the stuttering history and imaging findings should allow the disorders to be distinguished.
- Local infiltration from tumours or granulomatous disease.
- *Facial onset sensory motor neuropathy (FOSMN)* is a newly described, and apparently very rare, condition which presents with trigeminal sensory loss progressing to sensory disturbance in the upper limbs, a pattern mimicking syringobulbia. Wasting, weakness, and fasciculation of the tongue lead to MND being considered, and patients go on to develop respiratory muscle weakness. Immunomodulatory therapy has no effect and FOSMN is considered to be a neurodegenerative disorder. Upper motor neuron signs are absent and the pathology of motor neuron degeneration in this disorder is distinct from MND.

Infections

- HIV can occasionally cause an MND-like syndrome. Patients are typically younger than the MND age group, and have a rapid progression with extramotor neurological dysfunction and an inflammatory CSF examination. Some patients respond to combination anti-retroviral therapy (HAART).
- Previous infection with poliovirus is still common worldwide. Therefore a small proportion of sporadic ALS patients will coincidentally have suffered from polio in earlier life. Post-polio muscular atrophy (PPMA) occurs many years after the acute attack of poliomyelitis and is multifactorial in origin. Age-dependant loss of motor function and co-morbidities such as degenerative arthritis may contribute. Some patients undoubtedly show neurophysiological evidence of acute-on-chronic denervation. There is no evidence to support the hypothesis that PPMA is due to reactivation of latent poliovirus. The disorder is very slowly progressive and not life threatening (see Post-polio syndrome, Chapter 14).
- Other viruses such as West Nile and Japanese B have been reported to occasionally cause lower motor neuron involvement.
- HTLV I associated myelopathy ('tropical spastic paraparesis) is endemic in Japan, the Caribbean, South America, and elsewhere, HTLV I usually causes a slowly progressive myelopathy with early bladder involvement, but there have been occasional reports of mixed upper and lower motor neuron syndromes. In endemic areas it is self-evident that there will be patients with typical MND who are coincidentally positive for HTLV I and a causal relationship should not be assumed.
- Lyme disease is a controversial cause of an MND-like syndrome. Most cases have not been substantiated, but the possibility of an association has received much publicity and will therefore be raised from time to time by MND patients. The typical features of neurological Lyme disease are polyradiculopathy or meningoencephalitis, and the vast majority of *Borrelia burgdorferi* infections are believed to be self-limiting.

Radiation myeloneuropathy

Although modern radiotherapy regimes have been modified to avoid damage to neurological tissue, the long latency of this process means that occasional patients present decades after initial treatment.

- Upper limb: brachial plexopathy leading to weakness and wasting of the upper limb occurs after radiotherapy for breast cancer. Pain is a prominent feature and, with an appropriate history, MND is unlikely to be a major consideration.
- Lower limb: radiotherapy to the pelvis and para-aortic lymph nodes for testicular and gynaecological tumours is associated with a lower motor neuron syndrome in which sensory symptoms and signs can be very modest. The latency to developing symptoms may be decades and therefore the history of exposure may need to be specifically sought. The condition is usually slowly progressive and may undergo periods of arrest.

Inclusion body myositis

This disorder is rarer than MND. Weakness, typically of distal upper limb flexors, progresses very slowly over several years. Quadriceps wasting is also a typical feature. Dysphagia may occasionally occur. The confusion with MND arises because the EMG may show neurogenic change. Muscle biopsy is usually required to confirm the diagnosis.

Pure motor demyelinating neuropathies

- Chronic inflammatory demyelinating polyneuropathy (CIDP) is typically a symmetrical sensorimotor neuropathy affecting the legs more than the arms which is unlikely to be confused with MND.
- However, a small percentage of patients with demyelinating neuropathy can have a pure motor variant, usually also symmetrical and proximal. On investigation:
  - Reduced motor conduction velocity (and sometimes conduction block) can be detected on neurophysiology.
  - Lumbar puncture may show a raised protein.
- The more specific entity of multifocal motor neuropathy (MMN) with conduction block has characteristic clinical features:
  - Younger age of onset than MND: 80% of patients present between 20 and 50 years of age.
  - Slowly progressive, asymmetrical or unilateral weakness of the distal upper limb, with a predilection for wrist and finger extension.
  - Striking lack of wasting in weak muscles, except late in disease.
  - Cranial nerve involvement rare, respiratory involvement very rare.
  - CSF protein not usually raised.
  - Conduction block, i.e. failure of a nerve impulse to propagate through an intact axon, can be detected as a drop in CMAP amplitude on proximal v distal nerve stimulation.
  - In contrast to CIDP, worsens with steroid treatment.
  - Responds to intravenous immunoglobulin.

Fasciculation syndromes

The presence of fasciculation in the absence of wasting, weakness, or upper motor neuron signs presents a potentially difficult problem. However some general guidelines can be applied:

- A very small fraction of patients who ultimately turn out to have MND present with isolated fasciculations as the first symptom, weakness being a much commoner complaint. Therefore most patients presenting with isolated fasciculations to neurological clinics have benign fasciculations, and can be reassured without the need for EMG.

● There is no evidence that a prior history of benign fasciculations is a risk factor for developing MND. Fasciculation that persists for more than a year without the development of weakness or other objective neurological signs is unlikely to be due to MND.

● Benign fasciculations are in general more intrusive than pathological fasciculations, but characteristically come and go and are exacerbated by psychological stress, caffeine, exercise and post-alcohol. Pathological fasciculations are more persistent over months and tend to occur whatever the background factors.

● Fasciculation of the tongue is, for practical purposes, never a benign phenomenon. However, it is important to examine the tongue relaxed in the floor of the mouth, as tongue tremor can be easily mistaken for fasciculation by the inexperienced.

● The recent onset of cramps, in patients presenting with fasciculation, should raise the suspicion of MND.

● Conditions other than MND in which fasciculations may be prominent include:
  • cramp-fasciculation syndrome (worth checking for anti K$^+$-channel antibodies)
  • Kennedy's disease (see Chapter 14)
  • conduction block neuropathies
  • compressive radiculopathy.

Spinal muscular atrophies

For a full discussion of individual diseases see Chapter 14. Spinal muscular atrophies are a diverse group of mainly genetic conditions characterised by pure lower motor neuron degeneration. They are usually associated with a family history, are symmetrical and slowly progressive, and have characteristic patterns of distribution, which in general mean they should not be confused with MND.

Conveying the diagnosis of motor neuron disease

The person conveying a serious diagnosis like MND should:

- Be an expert in the diagnosis of neurological disease, so that diagnostic error is kept to a minimum.
- Be in a position to devote adequate time to the consultation without interruption.
- Have all available information to hand, including the results of investigations.
- Be sufficiently knowledgeable about the disease to answer the initial questions that arise.
- Be able to convey complex concepts in a way that can be understood by patients.
- Have rapid access to people and structures to support the patient and have a clear plan for onward management.

Research has demonstrated that an unduly negative experience at the time of diagnosis can have lasting psychological impact as the disease progresses. The following guidelines have emerged from qualitative studies of the process of breaking bad news:

- The diagnosis should always be conveyed in person and never by phone or mail.
- A quiet environment without interruption is important. Mobile phones and pagers should be switched off.
- The patient should be supported by a close relative or friend and by a non-physician health care professional (e.g. a nurse).
- An initial attempt should be made to understand what the patient already knows.
- A clear statement should be made that the problem is a serious one, as a warning that bad news is coming and a prelude to specifically mentioning the diagnosis.
- The approach should be 'patient-centred', i.e. individualized and sensitive to the patient's educational, and cultural background. Verbal and non-verbal cues should be used to understand how much the patient actually wants to know.
- Each patient has a different capacity to absorb information and this should be given at a rate appropriate for the individual.
- Frequent checks should be made to assess that the patient has absorbed what has been said and is ready for more information.
- Euphemisms should be avoided and the terms 'motor neuron disease' or 'amyotrophic lateral sclerosis' should be used explicitly and unambiguously and then explained, in terms which the patient can understand.
- There is no absolute rule about how much information to convey at the time of diagnosis. This depends on responding to each patient as an individual and answering their questions honestly, but not brutally.

- Patients who have some knowledge of the disease are likely to be aware of the most challenging aspects of MND through high profile media cases and publicity surrounding physician-assisted suicide. A balanced but honest view of the natural history of MND should be offered. It is reasonable to point out that none of the collective features of MND are inevitable in every case. For example, significant numbers of patients communicate normally throughout their illness.
- Emphasize that the disease is variable and that each person is on an individual journey. Unqualified statements about the 'average survival' being 2–3 years are likely to be misunderstood as 'the doctor gave me 2 years to live'. A better approach is to explain simply that there are some patients who live for much longer than average and that more time is needed to establish the rate of change.
- Patients who are already aware of the disease fear 'choking to death' and it is important to identify this concern and to offer reassurance that this does not occur.
- Explain that there is a plan of assessment and management, that the symptoms of MND can be treated, and that the patient will be offered support and will not be abandoned.
- If possible the contact details of the local specialist support nurse and for the relevant MND patient support group should be given to the patient.
- We have found that patients and relatives appreciate a tape recording of the initial consultation where the diagnosis and its implications are explained. Studies from the cancer field support this approach.
- A follow up appointment within a few days is ideal.

References and further reading

Beghi E, Millul A, Micheli A, Vitelli E, Logroscino G for the SLALOM Group (2007). Incidence of ALS in Lombardy, Italy. *Neurology*, 68, 141–145.

Forbes RB, Colville S, Cran GW, Swingler RJ (2004). Scottish Motor Neurone Disease Register. Unexpected decline in survival from amyotrophic lateral sclerosis/motor neurone disease. *J Neurol Neurosurg Psychiatry*, 75, 1753–5.

Haverkamp LJ, Appel V, Appel SH (1995). Natural history of amyotrophic lateral sclerosis in a database population. *Brain*, 118, 707–719.

Logroscino G, Traynor BJ, Hardiman O et al. (2008). Descriptive epidemiology of amyotrophic lateral sclerosis: new evidence and unsolved issues. *J Neurol Neurosurg Psychiatry*, 79, 6–11.

Natural history of motor neuron disease

The taxonomy of MND

MND can be regarded as a 'syndrome' comprising a range of clinical phenotypes, with the common theme of a progressive degenerative motor neuronopathy. The justification for considering these phenotypes as part of the same disease entity is that: (a) they all share common pathological features; (b) any of the phenotypes can occur as part of familial MND with mutations in the same gene; (c) initial atypical presentations often progress to a more generalized ALS clinical picture. Sub-division can be made on clinical grounds, according to different criteria which are not mutually exclusive:

• relative degree of UMN or LMN involvement: ALS, PMA and PLS
• diffuse or regional distribution, e.g. flail arm, bulbar (PBP)
• rates of progression: rapid and slow
   • 'referral paradox': reduced interval from symptom onset to diagnosis is a surrogate marker of rapid progression and poor prognosis
• age at onset: younger (<45) versus older
• cognitive involvement: frank FTD versus minor degrees of loss of executive function
• familial or sporadic.

Definition by UMN/LMN involvement

This analysis is the traditional method of sub-dividing MND clinico-pathologically. It is likely that there are two concurrent disease processes occurring in MND   one within the corticospinal tract and one at the anterior horn cells, summating to form a clinical spectrum with a continuous distribution:

• Mixed (Amyotrophic Lateral Sclerosis, ALS):
   • ~80% of cases
   • UMN (corticospinal tract, seen as 'lateral sclerosis', or gliosis, of the spinal cord neuropathologically)
   • LMN (anterior horn cell death leading to muscle wasting, termed amyotrophy)
   • 'typical' or Charcot-type Amyotrophic Lateral Sclerosis (ALS)
   • frequently used synonymously with the term 'MND'.
• LMN-predominant:
   • 5–15% of cases
   • only wasting (LMN signs)
   • no clear UMN signs detectable clinically (but may be pathologically)
   • termed Progressive Muscular Atrophy (PMA) in pure form.
• UMN-predominant:
   • ~2–3% of cases
   • UMN-only signs
   • no detectable wasting clinically (evidence of denervation may be found on EMG)
   • termed Primary Lateral Sclerosis (PLS) in pure form (at least 4 years without detectable LMN signs).

Regional phenotypes

These are defined by predominant body region involved:
- flail arm/leg
- Progressive Bulbar Palsy (PBP)
- respiratory-onset

Rates of progression

Arbitrary definition which cuts across other phenotypic classifications:
- Rapid (<2 years from symptom onset):
  - early respiratory involvement
  - bulbar-onset disease
  - A4V *SOD1* gene carriers
  - basophilic-inclusion disease (pathological diagnosis – often young females, more frequent in Japanese).
- Slow (>10 years from symptom onset):
  - PLS
  - D90A *SOD1* gene homozygotes
  - younger age at onset (<45).

Age at onset

Mean age at onset is ~65 years in both men and women.
- Young onset (<45):
  - generally slower progression
  - more likely to have a genetic origin
  - juvenile genetic forms (ALS2) may resemble PLS.
- Older onset:
  - generally faster progression
  - multiple co-morbidities contribute to poor outcome
  - more prevalent bulbar-onset in elderly females.

Cognitive involvement

MND has a clear clinical, genetic and pathological overlap with fronto-temporal dementia (FTD), and the two 'pure' conditions can be considered at two ends of a clinico-pathological spectrum (see Neuropathology, Chapter 1):
- Mild cognitive impairment:
  - detectable in at least 30% of MND patients
  - predominantly executive dysfunction
  - reduced verbal fluency the most consistent abnormality.
  Frank FTD
  - <5% of established MND patients
  - family history more common
  - occasionally precedes onset of MND
  - generally faster progression
  - ubiquitinated TDP-43 inclusions neuropathologically.

Familial or sporadic

Approximately 5% of patients give a history of a first degree relative who also suffered from MND. There is a small, but finite, chance that a rare disease like MND might occur in two family members by chance.

However, two members of a family with MND is usually indicative of a genetic basis for the disease (see Chapter 6).
- Familial MND:
  - Indistinguishable on purely clinical grounds from sporadic MND.
  - Family history may be incomplete and some members may be mislabelled with 'multiple sclerosis' or dementia.
  - Median age of onset is 10 years younger than sporadic disease.
  - Wide range of survival.
  - Variable penetrance leading to 'skipping of generations' may occur.

Amyotrophic lateral sclerosis

This represents at least 80% of all MND cases. Fundamental to the diagnosis is progressive motor weakness with mixed UMN and LMN signs. Median survival is 30 months from symptom onset, with the following typical features:

- History:
  - Arm, leg, or bulbar onset (approximately equal).
  - Patients report weakness, clumsiness, stiffness, or wasting.
  - Generally ipsilateral before contralateral limb spread.
  - No prominent sensory symptoms.
  - No prominent sphincter symptoms.
  - Gender ratio 3:2 male:female.
  - Wide variation in age of onset (mean mid-60s).
- Examination:
  - Prominent wasting, but UMN-predominant as well as LMN-predominant forms exist.
  - Usually visible fasciculations (rarely intrusive to patient).
  - Hyper-reflexia in the presence of local wasting.
  - May show frankly pathological reflexes, e.g. Hoffman, and sometimes corticobulbar reflexes, e.g. brisk jaw jerk, facial jerks, glabellar tap.
  - Plantar responses often extensor (not essential).
  - May demonstrate emotional lability.
  - No prominent sensory abnormalities.
- Course:
  - Survival usually <5 years from symptom onset.
  - Respiratory involvement may be early or late in course, with prognosis generally poor when early.
  - Bulbar-onset generally associated with shorter survival (1–2 years).
  - At least 80% of patients develop clinically significant bulbar involvement (but it is not inevitable).
- Potential mimics:
  - Rare and over-stated in the literature.
  - Cervical spondylotic myeloradiculopathy.
  - Paraneoplastic neuromuscular syndromes.

Progressive muscular atrophy

The notion of a pure LMN form of MND remains controversial due to the neuropathological evidence of sub-clinical UMN involvement in many cases. Clinical case series vary widely in estimating the proportion of MND which is PMA, reflecting a lack of consensus criteria and that PMA often progresses to become 'LMN-predominant ALS'. In its 'pure' form, PMA is probably less than 5% of all MND and typically has the following features:

- History:
  - Always limb onset (arm=leg).
  - Patients report weakness, clumsiness, or wasting.
  - Generally ipsilateral before contralateral limb spread or spread to contralateral limb of the same region (i.e. bilateral arm or leg weakness).
  - No prominent sensory symptoms.
  - No prominent sphincter symptoms.
  - Gender ratio 2:1 male:female.
  - Wide variation in age of onset (mean mid-50s).
- Examination:
  - Prominent wasting.
  - Usually visible fasciculations.
  - Reduced or absent reflexes.
  - Plantar responses can be flexor, 'mute', or occasionally extensor
  - No prominent sensory abnormalities.
- Course:
  - Survival usually <4 years from symptom onset unless 'Flail arm/leg' (see Flail arm/leg syndrome, p. 44).
  - Respiratory involvement may be early or late in course and is a poor prognostic sign, especially when early.
  - At least 50% of patients develop bulbar involvement.
- Potential mimics:
  - Multi-focal Motor Neuropathy with Conduction Block.
  - Paraneoplastic neuropathy.
  - X-linked Spinobulbar Muscular Atrophy (Kennedy's syndrome).
  - Adult-onset Spinal Muscular Atrophy.
  - Chronic lead poisoning.
  - Porphyria.
  - Post-polio syndrome.

Primary lateral sclerosis

This diagnosis also attracts controversy because of the disparity between neurophysiological and clinical detection of LMN involvement, and uncertainty about the distinction between PLS and 'upper motor neuron-predominant ALS'. PLS, in essence an ascending spastic tetraparesis, accounts for only 2–3% of all MND and typically has the following features:

History:
- Time from symptom onset to formal diagnosis >4 years (by definition).
- Most frequently leg onset, insidious.
- Patients report stiffness, weakness, or clumsiness.
- Usually symmetrical limb involvement, e.g. paraparesis.
- No prominent sensory symptoms.
- Mild sphincter symptoms common, e.g. urinary frequency.
- Gender ratio 3:2 male:female.
- Narrow range of age of onset (mean early-50s).

Examination:
- No visible wasting or fasciculations (no denervation on EMG).
- Hyper-reflexia – usually widespread and symmetrical.
- Pathological reflexes common, e.g. Hoffman, brisk jaw jerk, facial jerks, glabellar tap.
- Plantar responses usually extensor.
- Emotional lability common.
- No prominent sensory abnormalities.
- Cognitive involvement rare.

Course:
- Survival usually >10 years from symptom onset.
- Majority of patients develop corticobulbar involvement.
- Respiratory involvement usually late.
- Late Parkinsonian features occasionally seen.

Potential mimics:
- Spinal cord compression.
- Hereditary Spastic Paraparesis.
- Primary Progressive Multiple Sclerosis.
- Progressive Supranuclear Palsy.
- Paraneoplastic encephalomyelopathy.

Mills' syndrome

This is a rare entity of 'progressive hemiplegia' that falls within the spectrum of PLS (<0.5% of MND cases overall). Typically features include:
- progressive spastic hemiplegia
- usually leg then ipsilateral arm
- widespread symmetrical hyper-reflexia
- no sensory findings
- occasionally subtle focal wasting but without fasciculations
- slow but relentless progression.

Flail arm/leg syndrome

These phenotypes fall within the PMA group, but are separated by their markedly slower progression in comparison to other PMA or ALS cases. They are defined by the following features:

Flail arm

- Up to 10% of all MND cases.
- Gender ratio possibly as great as 9:1 male:female in 'pure' form.
- Symmetrical, usually proximal upper limb disease (but distal upper limb predominant ALS may fall within this category when it is slowly progressive).
- LMN features predominate – flaccid wasting and hypo-reflexia.
- UMN signs may be found incidentally in the legs, but weakness largely confined to upper limbs.
- 50% develop bulbar symptoms but not marked.
- Survival 5–10 years from onset.
- Synonyms for flail arm MND:
  - Brachial diplegia
  - 'Man in a barrel' syndrome
  - Vulpian-Bernhardt syndrome.

Flail leg

This group is less well defined:
- Approximately 5% of all MND cases.
- Occasionally termed Patrikios' disease or the 'pseudopolyneuritic form of MND'.
- Gender ratio 2:1 male:female.
- Unilateral or symmetrical distal leg weakness at onset.
- LMN features predominate – flaccid wasting and hypo-reflexia.
- UMN signs may be found incidentally elsewhere, but weakness largely confined to lower limbs.
- Progressively ascends to involve the arms.
- Bulbar involvement less common.
- Survival 5–7 years from onset.

Progressive bulbar palsy

A clinical term with arbitrarily defined features:
- ~5% of all MND cases.
- Gender ratio estimate 1:3 male:female; generally older patients.
- Bulbar onset with relative confinement of disease to this region (perhaps for at least 1 year).
- Variably mixed LMN/UMN features.
- There may be rapid progression to complete anarthria, but then an apparent period of relative stabilization (the 'ambulant anarthrics').
- Overall survival still usually <2 years, with a range of 6 months to 4 years.
- Early PEG improves survival.
- Early familiarity with communication devices helpful e.g. Lightwriter®.

The term 'bulbar-onset' ALS is, to some extent, an unsatisfactory piece of shorthand. It does not denote one condition with a unified prognosis. Patients with PBP as described above can have a slow progression with disease isolated to one region for a prolonged period. Patients with bulbar-onset ALS, by which is meant bulbar involvement as part of a more generalized picture involving the limbs, have early respiratory involvement and, on average, a poor prognosis.

Respiratory-onset MND

- ~2% of all MND cases.
- Gender ratio 3:1 male:female.
- Symptoms (may be nebulous initially):
  - exertional dyspnoea
  - orthopnoea
  - poor cough
  - sleep fragmentation
  - lack of sleep refreshment
  - early morning headache
  - excessive day-time somnolence.
- There may be raised serum bicarbonate.
- Arterial blood gas confirms hypercapnoea.
- Early NIV improves symptoms dramatically and also has a modest effect on survival.
- Overall survival 2–3 years (i.e. similar to typical ALS).

Extramotor and other unusual manifestations of MND

The concept of MND as a pure motor disease has broken down in recent years with the realization that selective vulnerability of motor neurons is relative.

Parkinsonism: pathological studies have demonstrated reduced neurons in the substantia nigra in ALS, but not Lewy bodies. Some sporadic ALS patients develop mild to moderate extrapyramidal rigidity, but it is usually not the main cause of their disability. There is no evidence that l-dopa is a useful treatment in this situation.

Autonomic features: patients frequently observe minor changes which might suggest autonomic dysfunction such as excessive sweating, bladder and bowel dysfunction, and poor peripheral circulation. However, in each case there are other potential explanations. Bladder spasticity can lead to urinary urgency and frequency, immobility promotes constipation, and peripheral vasomotor tone is reduced in a paralysed limb from any cause. Laboratory testing can reveal mild, sub-clinical involvement of the autonomic nervous system. Sudden unexpected death certainly occurs in a small proportion of patients and this could be due to cardiac autonomic dysfunction, but this is very difficult to prove.

Sensory involvement: it is not uncommon for patients to describe their experience of progressive paralysis of limbs in sensory terms such as 'deadness' or 'numbness', but careful history taking usually leads to the conclusion that this is a figure of speech. Neurophysiological studies (SSEPs) have suggested that sub-clinical involvement of sensory pathways is common. Identification of objective sensory signs should always prompt a reconsideration of the diagnosis, however.

Altered smell and taste are common in other neurodegenerative diseases but seem to be rare in MND. Riluzole has occasionally been associated with loss of taste.

Further reading

Wijesekera LC, Mathers S, et al. (2009). Natural history and clinical features of the flail arm and flail leg ALS variants. Neurology, 72, 1087–94.

Shoesmith CL, Findlater K, Rowe A, Strong MJ (2007). Prognosis of amyotrophic lateral sclerosis with respiratory onset. J Neurol Neurosurg Psychiatry, 78, 629–31.

Organization of MND services

Background

MND is a complex disease and the expert driven multidisciplinary care team model is widely accepted as the ideal. Outside of the context of the tertiary referral clinical neuroscience centre, MND is a relatively rare disease, and forms a small part of the workload of most health care professionals. Prior to the establishment of specialist clinics, care was fragmented, patchy in coverage, and not always delivered in a timely fashion.

- The advantages of specialist MND care clinics:
  - Specialists can develop their expertise to the advantage of patients. There are still relatively few neurologists in the UK by European and North American standards. UK neurologists in district general hospitals can expect to see 4–6 new patients per year with MND. This is an adequate number to remain competent in the diagnosis of the disease, but it would take a lifetime of practice to develop a good working knowledge of MND in all of its clinical manifestations.
  - There is evidence from some countries (Ireland and Italy) that specialist care improves survival. However, such studies are difficult to perform without significant biases that could distort conclusions about outcome. For example, patients motivated to travel to specialist centres may be different in a number of ways, not least in having less aggressive disease.
  - Patients can see a range of healthcare professionals in one visit.
  - Clinics can be patient-centred and organized on a flexible model rather than bound by the usual outpatient structure.
  - Care can be delivered locally but coordinated to maximum effect and with appropriate timeliness.
  - Patients can access the latest information about research and also participate, such as in clinical trials of new drugs.
  - Research into every aspect of the disease is facilitated.
  - People affected by MND can meet others in the same situation.
  - Specialist clinics can form national networks for integration of research and care.
  - Training of neurologists and paramedical specialists should improve through the dissemination of good practice.
  - More effective interaction with funding bodies and patient advocacy groups such as the MND Association in the UK.
- Some possible disadvantages:
  - Patients may have to travel great distances to attend a specialist clinic.
  - Some patients are put off by not wanting to encounter others with MND at a more advanced stage.
  - If all the expertise is concentrated at the centre, doctors and therapists at the periphery may become deskilled by lack of familiarity with the disease. Although most primary diagnoses of MND will continue to made by generalist neurologists, these doctors may not develop the expertise gained by following the disease through its complete course.
  - It may be difficult for the centre to direct the provision of local services from a distance.

The MND Care Centre Programme in the UK demonstrates how specialist services have evolved in recent decades. Since 1990 the MND Association has supported the development of a network of care centres throughout England, Wales, and Northern Ireland. These have mainly been established at regional neuroscience departments. There are currently 17 care centres. The care centre model is flexible in its structure and each care centre is unique in the way it is organized and managed, reflecting local resources. The care centres are united by adhering to the MNDA Standards of Care charter which sets benchmarks for access and referral times.

In traditional models of medical care, individual medical specialists are usually seen as having very distinct roles:

- Neurologists: primary providers of assessment, diagnosis, and management of disease.
- Rehabilitation specialists: primary providers of therapy, equipment, social/psychological support, and service coordination.
- Palliative care consultants: providers of terminal care, management of death, and bereavement.

These divisions may be entirely appropriate in many circumstances and the initial diagnosis of MND certainly remains the preserve of the neurologist. It is also more likely that MND clinics based in regional neuroscience centres will be directed by academic neurologists with an active research program, and many patients greatly appreciate the opportunity to participate in research. However, the nature of MND is such as to promote a more flexible interchange between the three domains of neurology, rehabilitation, and palliative care. Many neurologist-led MND clinics offer coordinated care throughout the disease to the end of life. Even if the most common model for care of MND patients is neurologist led, there are alternative approaches which can be equally effective. What matters most to patients is that they have rapid, timely, and ongoing access to a group of specialists who are interested in their problems and have the necessary skills to help them.

The MND Clinical Care Team

Structure
- The structure and membership of specialist care teams may vary depending on local factors. The individuals listed below might all be present in one clinical area and see patients at one visit, or may act as a 'virtual team' and see patients in their own clinics but under coordinated arrangements. The MND care team typically consists of:
  - Neurologist.
  - Specialist Nurse.
  - Occupational Therapist (OT).
  - Dietitian.
  - Speech and Language Therapist.
  - Physiotherapist.
  - Respiratory specialist nurse.
  - Enteral feeding/endoscopy specialist nurse.
  - Clinical Psychologist.
  - Association Visitors.

Specific roles of individual team members
This is described according to the UK MNDA Care Centre model but the roles outlined below are equally applicable to MND clinics in other settings such as palliative care.
- Neurologist:
  - Director of care centre and team leadership.
  - Initial diagnosis and provision of second opinions for other colleagues.
  - Classification of disease according to subtype and rate of progression in order to help other team members prioritise care.
  - Ongoing expert advice during the disease course.
  - Direct link with GP.
  - Research and education.
- Care-centre coordinator/Specialist Nurse:
  - Coordination of clinic.
  - Monitoring of ALSFRS and other measures of disease progression.
  - Single point of contact for patients (e.g. available by pager and a dedicated email address).
  - Advice and support to families and carers affected by MND.
  - Link with community-based services.
  - Links with MND Association.
  - Education and dissemination of good practice.
- Occupational Therapist:
  - Monitoring posture.
  - Advice about special equipment such as collars.
  - Assessing the need for and facilitating provision of wheelchairs and linking to local wheelchair services.
  - Links with community OTs who can visit patients at home.
  - Education and dissemination of good practice.

- Dietitian:
  - Monitor patients' nutritional status.
  - Advice about diet to maximise nutritional status and prevent problems during eating for patients with bulbar symptoms.
  - Planning of timely interventions such as PEG.
  - Links with community-based dietitians.
  - Liaison with ward-based staff if patients are admitted.
  - Education and dissemination of good practice.
- Speech and Language Therapist:
  - Monitor speech and swallowing.
  - Advice about exercises to improve clarity and prevent choking episodes.
  - Assessment for different types of augmented communication aids.
  - Links with community specialists.
  - Education and dissemination of good practice.
- Physiotherapist (see Chapter 11):
  - Advice about exercises and stretching programmes to manage cramps and spasticity and minimise secondary disability from contractures.
  - Monitoring walking and balance and advice about preventing falls.
  - Provision of equipment such as walking sticks, crutches and splints.
  - Breathing exercises such as breath stacking and assisted cough techniques.
  - Education and dissemination of good practice.
- Respiratory specialist nurse:
  - Monitors lung function (FVC, SNP etc.).
  - Sleep Questionnaire.
  - Coordination of overnight oximetry.
  - Expertise in detection of early signs of respiratory failure.
  - Direct links with respiratory medicine team for provision of Non Invasive Ventilation (NIV) as appropriate.
  - Education and dissemination of good practice.
- Enteral-feeding specialist nurse :
  - Coordinates with MND team about timely insertion of PEG.
  - Education of patient, family, and carers.
  - Links with ward staff, endoscopy team, and community-based teams.
  - Education and dissemination of good practice.
- Clinical Psychologist:
  - Helps patients with adjustment following diagnosis.
  - Cognitive behavioural therapy for patients with panic attacks or other severe adjustment reactions.
  - Assessment and differential diagnosis of apparent cognitive impairment.
  - Advice about capacity to consent.
  - Advice and support to families caring for people with FTD.
  - Education and dissemination of good practice.
- Volunteers from the MNDA:
  - Greet patients in clinic.
  - Introduce patients and families to their local MND branch.

- Advice and support to patient and families.
- Links with other sources of help such as home visitors.

Liaison with community-based health care professionals

Much of the care that really makes a difference to the lives of patients with MND is delivered in the community and not a regional neuroscience centre. It is important to consider the following:

- The perspective of those directing the resources available for the management of disability outside of the acute hospital setting may be quite different from the MND specialist team.
- Their resources are often limited and there are many competing demands from a range of problems in addition to MND.
- The role of the specialist clinic team is to ensure that social services and community-based health care professionals understand the nature of MND, the often rapid rate of progression, and the role and limitations of the specialist clinic as a provider of care.
- There may come a point in the disease trajectory when the patient no longer wishes to travel to a specialist clinic. It is critical that the appropriate structures are then in place to enable the patient to benefit from the support of their community team.

There are a number of ways in which specialist clinics can link with their local MNDA branches. They may jointly run the following:

- Friends and family support groups which provide an opportunity for mutual support through regular meetings, discussion groups, theatre trips, social evenings, etc.
- Carers' groups: a forum for carers to get together to talk and learn from shared experiences.
- Educational programmes and study days.
- Fund raising.

Role of the general practitioner

- The average GP in the UK has a list size of 2000–2500 patients.
- On a per capita basis it might therefore be predicted that an average GP would encounter a new diagnosis of MND once in their professional lifetime.
- Modern health centres typically consist of 5–10 GPs working as a cooperative group. At any one time such a practice may have no patients with MND at all or at most 1–2 at a time.
- It should therefore be self-evident that a complex disease like MND is potentially very challenging for GPs.
- People living with MND often have unrealistic expectations of what their GP ought to know about the disease. The initial diagnosis may have been delayed in many cases and this tends to elevate the status of the hospital specialist, who may be seen by patients as the source of all solutions to the problems that MND raises.
- It is critical that GPs are involved in the ongoing care of MND patients at all stages of their disease and that specialist centres discourage excessive dependency on their services, which are, by the nature of outpatient care, often inaccessible out of office hours.
- The GP has the important perspective of having known the patient before the diagnosis of MND, will have a better understanding of the effect of MND in the context of the patient's past medical history, and will often have a much better appreciation of the impact of the disease on the whole family.
- GPs in the UK hold the drug budget and take the prime responsibility for prescribing, and it is therefore critical that all drug treatment decisions made in the hospital setting are made in partnership with the GP and that lines of communication are efficient.
- The effective involvement of community-based nurses ('district nurses') who are attached to health centres depends on GPs.
- GPs often control access to community hospital facilities which provide an important source of respite care and access to community physiotherapy and OT.
- Most MND patients wish to have their end-of-life care in their own home (see Chapter 12). This can only be successful if the GP is fully engaged in the patient's care from an early stage and is aware of any advanced decisions to refuse treatment.

Rehabilitation medicine

In the recent past, when neurologists saw themselves as primarily providing a diagnostic service but not offering ongoing care to patients with chronic neurological disease, neurorehabilitation services took on much of the management of MND, although there was marked variation in what was available. In some regions this is still the model employed and, providing there is an efficient care pathway between neurology and rehabilitation, is a highly effective mechanism for MND care. In our practice there is a close partnership with neurorehabilitation services, with frequent interchange of junior medical staff, and a number of our paramedical specialists work jointly between the MND clinic and neurorehabilitation. Particular indications for referral to a specialist neurorehabilitation service include:

- Complex disability management, especially in the context of slowly progressive MND where long term solutions are required and periods of stable but severe disability can be anticipated. This might include:
  - Assessment for and provision of augmentative and alternative communication aids (AACs).
  - Environmental control systems.
  - Specialist seating and posture management.
  - Mobile arm supports.
  - Preparation for long-term residential care.
- Multidisciplinary management of spasticity including botulinum toxin therapy, intrathecal baclofen pumps, etc.
- Access to highly specialist therapists with particular skills not routinely available in the acute hospital setting:
  - Clothing adviser.
  - Advice about driving and vehicle adaptation.
  - Psychological help for children and families.
  - Sexual therapists.
- Short periods of intensive assessment and therapy, so that the person with MND can return to their home with a number of complex problems addressed at a single time point.

Palliative care specialists

- Although, historically, palliative care medicine developed as a speciality around the hospice movement, the services and expertise they offer now extends into acute hospital settings and domiciliary care.
- The caseload in palliative care medicine has in the past been dominated by cancer, but there is now widespread recognition of the need for palliative care specialists to engage in the management of progressive neurological, especially neurodegenerative, diseases.
- In some areas palliative care services are involved early after diagnosis and become the primary MDT managing MND.
- As long as there is a clear emphasis on enablement and symptom control most patients will not interpret this as irrelevant to their needs at a time when they do not perceive themselves to be in the terminal phase of the illness.
- Another common model is joint clinics with the palliative care specialist embedded as a member of the MDT.
- In the UK, the hospice movement has been at the forefront of advances in symptom control. Most neurologists do not have specific training or expertise in end-of-life care. Therefore, close liaison with a palliative care physician should be routine practice regardless of whether care is 'handed over' or shared.
- An important principle to convey to patients is that palliative care specialists do not just deal with the end of life but are experts in symptom control at any stage of the disease.
- Our own practice is dictated by flexibility and responsiveness to individual patient preference:
  - Patients who live alone are most likely to express feelings of anxiety about being cared for and find early contact with hospice comforting.
  - Others wish to have hospice care as an available option but plan to remain at home.
  - For some patients periods of respite care in a hospice are a critical way of relieving carer burden and maintaining the equilibrium of the home situation, which would otherwise break down.
  - Some patients consistently refuse contact with palliative care services despite our best efforts to emphasize the benefits.
- A minority of our patients deteriorate unexpectedly or their care situation breaks down and they are admitted to an acute neurology ward. Hospital-based palliative care specialists provide important expertise in this setting in facilitating symptom control in the terminal phase.

Further reading

MNDA (2004). *Standards of Care*. http://www.mndassociation.org/for_professionals/sharing_good_practice/standards_of.html

Measurement of change

Introduction

- Understanding the rate of change in motor neuron disease is critical for:
  - predicting overall prognosis
  - anticipating functional decline to plan disability management
  - conducting clinical trials
  - distinguishing different phenotypes.
- The ideal method of assessment should:
  - be sufficiently low-tech to be applicable in any clinical setting
  - provide an accurate measure of both upper and lower motor neuron dysfunction
  - reflect the disease burden relevant to the patient; for example, manual muscle testing may identify changes in muscle power which do not actually translate into change in specific functions recognized by patients
  - be tolerated by patients at any stage of their illness.; this is particularly important in clinical trials, where missing data as the disease progresses has serious consequences
  - have high inter-rater reliability
  - have a high predictive value for timing of interventions like NIV and PEG
  - allow accurate prediction of life expectancy.
- Survival is often used as an outcome measure in trials and natural history studies. Unfortunately it is not a totally unambiguous measure and may reflect factors other than the natural history of the disease:
  - It is affected by interventions such as enteral nutrition and NIV.
  - Invasive ventilation unequivocally prolongs the disease course.
  - For clinical trials it requires long term analysis to generate enough power to detect treatment differences.
- Current clinical trials are extremely expensive and typically require several hundred people in each arm to detect potential treatment effects. The development of sensitive measures of disease progression (e.g. using imaging) might allow drugs to be prescreened for biological effect before being entered into large scale trials, or allow a drastic reduction in the number of subjects needed to show a significant effect.

Manual muscle testing

Common sense would suggest that in a disease where loss of voluntary muscle action dominates the clinical picture longitudinal testing of individual muscle groups should represent a good marker of disease progression. However:

- In terms of disease management, testing of muscle power is much less informative than an assessment of functional impairment based around activities of daily living.
- In the setting of an MND care clinic the measurement of muscle power, while extremely informative for the neurologist in terms of natural history studies, may be demoralizing for the person with MND and simply serve as a statement of a decline of which they are all too aware.
- Even using established methods such as the MRC scale, there is still considerable variation in how muscle power is recorded.
- Some muscle groups are easier to test than others. For example, the standard neurological examination is biased towards the limbs and assessment of axial and pelvic muscles, which are important for stance and gait, are not examined in an objective way. Similarly, bulbar muscles are assessed in terms of function not strength.

Therefore, repetitive longitudinal muscle testing is mostly relevant to research settings, either in the context of a clinical trial or a formal natural history study. There are two types of muscle strength testing used in MND studies:

- Maximum voluntary isometric contraction (MVIC), in which muscle strength is measured using a specially constructed examination frame containing a type of strain gauge coupled to a computer for analysis. This is an accurate and highly reproducible method of measuring muscle weakness but has the obvious limitations of requiring specialized equipment, specially trained technicians, being time consuming, and of only being able to sample a limited number of muscles.
- Manual muscle testing (MMT) uses the MRC scale of muscle strength and produces a summated score, which can provide a longitudinal measure of disease progression, provided enough muscle groups are chosen. It has the advantage of not requiring specialized equipment and also of being part of the routine neurological examination and familiar to clinicians. However, it should be remembered that this is a non-linear (non-parametric) scale and the significance between any two different points on the scale is not constant. Despite this, parametric statistical tests are often misapplied to the MRC scale.

ALS Functional Rating Scale

Functional rating scales have the advantage in the clinic of being easy to apply and of reflecting aspects of the condition across a number of domains which are meaningful to patients. The ALSFRS has several advantageous features which mean that it is now the standard method of assessing disease progression in clinical trials and in MND clinics:

- It can be easily applied (even at a distance by phone contact).
- The scale has been validated as correlating with measures of muscle strength such as MVIC.
- It has internal consistency.
- There is evidence that the ALSFRS at clinical presentation is a predictor of overall survival, and groups of patients with lower scores at presentation also have a shorter latency from symptom onset to diagnosis, both reflecting more rapid disease progression.
- In the standard ALSFRS each of 10 domains is given a score of 0 to 4, with a total of 40.
- A revised version, taking into account respiratory function, has been devised and has 48 points on the scale (ALSFRS-R).

The use of ALSFRS for clinical trials is widespread but has the potential disadvantage of not being sufficiently sensitive to change to detect small effects.

Several other scales, in less widespread use, have been devised:

- Appel scale:
  - examines 5 domains (bulbar, respiratory, muscle strength, upper limb function, lower limb function)
  - a mixture of functional tests and questions, which potentially involves 4 separate assessors (neurologist, nurse, OT and respiratory) and takes 20 minutes.
- Norris scale and ALS severity scale were early attempts at assessment which have now largely been superseded.

The ALS Functional Rating Scale

1. Speech
4 Normal speech processes
3 Detectable speech disturbance
2 Intelligible with repeating
1 Speech combined with non-vocal communication
0 Loss of useful speech

2. Salivation
4 Normal
3 Slight but definite excess of saliva in mouth; may have nighttime drooling
2 Moderately excessive saliva; may have minimal drooling
1 Marked excess of saliva with some drooling
0 Marked drooling; requires constant tissue or handkerchief

3. Swallowing
4 Normal eating habits
3 Early eating problems – occasional choking
2 Dietary consistency changes
1 Needs supplemental tube feeding
0 NPO (exclusively parenteral or enteral feeding)

4. Handwriting
4 Normal
3 Slow or sloppy: all words are legible
2 Not all words are legible
1 Able to grip pen but unable to write
0 Unable to grip pen

5a. Cutting food and handling utensils (patients without gastrostomy)

4 Normal
3 Somewhat slow and clumsy, but no help needed
2 Can cut most foods, although clumsy and slow; some help needed
1 Food must be cut by someone, but can still feed slowly
0 Needs to be fed

5b. Cutting food and handling utensils (alternate scale for patients with gastrostomy)

4 Normal
3 Clumsy but able to perform all manipulations independently
2 Some help needed with closures and fasteners
1 Provides minimal assistance to caregiver
0 Unable to perform any aspect of task

6. Dressing and hygiene

4 Normal function
3 Independent and complete self-care with effort or decreased efficiency
2 Intermittent assistance or substitute methods
1 Needs attendant for self-care
0 Total dependence

7. Turning in bed and adjusting bed clothes

4 Normal
3 Somewhat slow and clumsy, but no help needed
2 Can turn alone or adjust sheets, but with great difficulty
1 Can initiate, but not turn or adjust sheets alone
0 Helpless

8. Walking

4 Normal
3 Early ambulation difficulties
2 Walks with assistance
1 Nonambulatory functional movement
0 No purposeful leg movement

9. Climbing stairs

4 Normal
3 Slow
2 Mild unsteadiness or fatigue
1 Needs assistance
0 Cannot do

10. Dyspnoea

4 None
3 Occurs when walking
2 Occurs with one or more: eating, bathing, dressing
1 Occurs at rest, either sitting or lying
0 Significant difficulty, considering mechanical support

11. Orthopnoea

4 None
3 Some difficulty sleeping, due to shortness of breath, doesn't routinely use >2 pillows
2 Needs extra pillows to sleep (>2)
1 Can only sleep sitting up
0 Unable to sleep

12. Respiratory insufficiency

4 None
3 Intermittent use of NIV
2 Continuous use of NIV at night
1 Continuous use of NIV day and night
0 Invasive mechanical ventilation

Forced vital capacity

Advantages of FVC as a measure of disease progression:
- Can be applied easily in the clinic setting with minimal training of clinic staff.
- Declines linearly as the disease progresses.
- Baseline FVC and the rate of decline predict survival.

Disadvantages:
- Requires the subject to be cooperative and to exert maximal effort.
- Some training is needed for the assessor to ensure the patient applies the correct technique.
- Percentage predicted FVC requires the height and other data to be available.
- There are significant technical limitations in patients with corticobulbar dysfunction.
- Its use as a primary outcome measure in clinical trials is still debated, although the slope of decline in FVC is becoming a standard measure.

Neurophysiology

The role of neurophysiology in the diagnosis of MND has been covered in Chapter 2. Given the importance of demonstrating motor neuron loss objectively at the time of diagnosis, is there a role for neurophysiology in assessing disease progress and providing prognostic information?

- The standard diagnostic neurophysiological examination is necessarily a sampling technique, rather than a systematic evaluation. In order to serve as a measure of disease progression, changes in neurophysiological parameters at individual sites must reflect the underlying disease progress in a fundamental sense. In general, EMG, decline in motor conduction velocity, and compound muscle action potential have not been useful in following the disease or providing accurate prognostic information.
- To justify techniques which are expensive, time-consuming, require special expertise and equipment, and expose the patient to discomfort, these must be demonstrated to be more sensitive to change than simple non-invasive clinical measures such as FVC and ALSFRS.

Motor unit number estimation (MUNE)

- This technique assesses lower motor neuron loss and requires the motor nerve to be stimulated at progressively lower levels until a threshold 'all or nothing' muscle response is obtained, which is taken to represent one motor unit. The intensity is then gradually increased so that subsequent motor units are recruited and recognized as quantal increases in the amplitude of muscle response. From the average amplitude of the individual motor units it is possible to estimate the total number of motor units from the maximal compound muscle action potential.
- A number of ways of estimating motor unit number are available and there is no gold-standard. More sophisticated statistical methods of calculating the mean size of motor units has improved the reliability of MUNE.
- MUNE has been used in clinical trials as a marker of progression and has performed as well as other standard measures. However, special training is required and rigorous criteria for test-retest reliability must be applied. While MUNE is likely to be used in future clinical trials, it has not found a place in routine clinical practice in assessing disease progression.

Transcranial magnetic stimulation (TMS)

- Assessment of upper motor neuron integrity can be achieved by applying a brief magnetic pulse over the motor cortex, which induces an electrical stimulus transmitted down the corticospinal tract.
- Recording over the limbs and subtraction of peripheral motor conduction time allows an estimate of central motor conduction time, and hence integrity of the corticospinal tract.
- Although useful as a research tool in understanding cortical hyperexcitability in the pathogenesis of MND, the technique is neither sensitive nor specific enough to be used in clinical practice.

Imaging

- A variety of imaging techniques have been investigated in MND but most are cross-sectional with mixed groups of patients, and relatively few attempts have been made to look at longitudinal markers of disease progression.
- Imaging of the brain has the obvious limitation that the spinal cord, the seat of much of the pathology in MND, is excluded. Therefore, it is only likely to be a meaningful method of following disease progression if the cerebral component of neuronal degeneration reflects some fundamental aspect of the disease as a whole.
- Diffusion imaging of the cord is in development.
- The burden of disability in MND, especially with the onset of respiratory features such as orthopnoea, limits the application of all imaging methods in later stages of the disease and makes longitudinal studies challenging.
- Disease heterogeneity means that large numbers of patients are needed to derive useful data. This is expensive and labour intensive.
- Despite these reservations, imaging offers one of the best prospects of identifying biomarkers of disease progression.

Structural MRI

- There are no specific correlates of disease progression associated with standard clinical MRI sequences and repeat scans are not indicated in routine clinical practice.
- T2 hyperintensity in the corticospinal tract occurs in a minority of patients (<40%). It may be a marker of more aggressive disease but this has not been systematically demonstrated.
- More sophisticated methods of structural imaging such as voxel-based morphometry, which compares atrophy in different brain regions, are still being assessed in ALS.

Magnetic resonance spectroscopy

- Uses ratios of creatine to phosphocreatine and creatine to choline to measure neuronal integrity.
- Can demonstrate damage in the motor cortex in MND.
- Has the potential advantage that it can be carried out on conventional clinical-grade MR scanners.
- Limitations include low spatial resolution and variable sensitivity to change over time.

Diffusion MRI

- The diffusion of water molecules in axons is non-random. This can be measured using MR indices such as fractional anisotropy (FA). Reductions in FA are an indirect measure of neuronal integrity.
- Probabilistic statistical methods can be used to compare FA in adjacent segments to reconstruct white matter tracts.
- Using diffusion tensor imaging (DTI) the integrity of the corticospinal tract can be measured.
- Many studies demonstrate that this can reliably detect patients with ALS and it has the potential to distinguish ALS from PLS.

Biomarkers

- A biomarker is an objective measure of an underlying biological process that can be used to measure disease progress and response to therapy.
- Both neurophysiology and imaging therefore have potential to act as biomarkers in MND.
- A number of attempts have been made to identify biomarkers in blood and CSF. Such approaches assume that the underlying pathological process in MND will be reflected in these tissue compartments. Although there is some evidence from research that CSF may contain factors directly relevant to the pathogenesis of motor neuron death, for blood this has not been established.
- Techniques where large-scale high-throughput analysis of gene expression (transcriptomics), protein expression (proteomics), and specific metabolites (metabolomics) can be combined may lead to advances in biomarker development.
- Identification of the 'ideal biomarker' in MND might lead to:
  - improved early diagnosis
  - better delineation of MND sub-types
  - assessment of disease progression
  - better prognostication
  - improved objectivity and sensitivity to change in clinical trials with lower numbers needed to show an effect.

Quality of life

Of the different things that could be assessed in MND, quality of life (QoL) is probably the most important to the person with the disease, but perhaps the most neglected by physicians. The clinical management of MND is necessarily focused on measuring decline in function in order to plan interventions and to prognosticate. Although good clinical teams will naturally focus on providing the best possible care for patients, it is rare for this to be formally measured in the course of an MND clinic.

- The impact of MND on the person with the disease, their family and carers, and society as a whole is not adequately described by the measurements outlined so far in this chapter. A more meaningful description of MND as a disease would be one which, in addition to loss of motor function, encompassed 'loss of personal biography'.
- Clinical trials focus on outcomes such as survival or rate of disease progression and often do not include sufficient assessment of whether the drug in question improves patients' well being. Given that new treatments are usually expensive, regulatory authorities are increasingly interested that investigators demonstrate an effect on QoL in drug trials so that therapies are 'cost effective'.
- There is preliminary evidence, supported by anecdotal clinical experience, that QoL, or at least psychological well-being, has a direct impact on survival.
- There is no validated MND-specific tool to assess QoL.
- Generic QoL scales that are frequently used in research studies, but not clinical practice, include:
  - SF-36
  - EuroQoL.
- Assessment of mood should be a standard part of MND care. The Beck depression inventory is a useful and rapid way of assessing depression.

Further reading

Turner MR, Kiernan MC, Leigh PN, Talbot K (2009). Biomarkers in amyotrophic lateral sclerosis. *Lancet Neurol*, 8, 94–109.

Cudkowicz M, Qureshi M, Shefner J (2004). Measures and markers in amyotrophic lateral sclerosis. *NeuroRx*, 1, 273–83.

Genetics of MND

Introduction to genetic neurological disease

Current estimates indicate that there are 21–23,000 genes in the human genome (www.ensembl.org). This is the same number for the mouse, chimpanzee, and other mammals, suggesting that biological complexity is not patterned primarily by the number of genes but by complex post-transcriptional and post-translational processing events. Variation at the nucleotide level (genotype) in combination with developmental events and environmental factors determines the manifestation of particular traits (phenotype). A significant proportion of all genetic disease have a neurological manifestation, either in isolation or as part of a complex multisystem disorder. Some of the limitations of genetic testing are outlined in Box 6.1.

Phenotype vs genotype

- A particular phenotype may be caused by mutations in different genes in different individuals. This is known as genetic heterogeneity. For example, hereditary spastic paraparesis, indistinguishable on clinical grounds, may be caused by mutations in paraplegin or spastin.
- A particular gene, mutated in different ways, may cause quite different phenotypes. For example, recessive mutations in the gene for senataxin cause 'ataxia with oculomotor apraxia Type I', whereas dominant mutations in senataxin cause ALS4 (see Familial amyotrophic lateral sclerosis (fALS)).

Types of mutation

- Chromosomal:
  - Abnormal number of chromosomes, e.g. trisomy-21 in Down's syndrome.
  - Large chromosomal deletions.
  - Microdeletions, increasingly recognized as a cause of non-syndromic mental retardation.
  - Ring chromosomes.
  - Translocations.
- Single base pair change:
  - Missense: results in an amino acid alteration in the translated protein.
  - Truncating: the base pair change creates a stop-codon.
  - A conservative change that does not alter the amino acid sequence but may alter splicing.
  - A non-coding change in an intron which alters splicing.
- Intragenic small-scale change:
  - Insertion of 1 or 2 base pairs, or 3 base pairs out of frame, may alter the reading frame of the mRNA to produce a 'nonsense' protein.
  - Insertion of a three base pair mutation in-frame will create a protein with an extra amino acid which is likely to have functional consequences.

- Dynamic mutations:
  - Triplet repeat disorders: these can be coding, such as the polyglutamine (CAG-repeat) diseases (Huntington's, spinocerebellar ataxia Types 1,2,3,6,7, X-linked SBMA), or non-coding, such as Fragile-X syndrome in which a massive CGG-trinucleotide repeat disrupts the promoter of the FMRP gene leading to transcriptional silencing.
  - Tetranucleotide repeat disorders, e.g. oculopharyngeal muscular dystrophy.
  - Dodecapeptide (Unverricht-Lundborg progressive myoclonic epilepsy).
- Copy number variation, e.g. duplication of PMP-22 leading to Charcot-Marie-Tooth disease Type 1a, triplication of alpha-synuclein leading to Parkinson's disease.

Box 6.1 Limitations of genetic testing

- Missense mutations may be spread throughout the gene requiring the whole gene to be sequenced exon by exon. This is time consuming and expensive.
- The extent to which non-coding mutations cause disease is largely unknown and these regions (introns, 5' and 3' untranslated regions) are not usually included in sequencing.
- Many genetic neurological diseases are rare and routine laboratory testing in unavailable. Research laboratories may offer testing but without a clear commitment or timescale or the same quality control that exists in clinical molecular genetics laboratories.

Some symbols used in pedigree drawing

The symbols commonly used in pedigree drawing are shown in Figure 6.1.

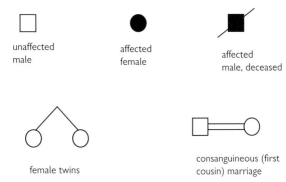

Fig. 6.1 Symbols used in pedigree drawing.

Patterns of genetic inheritance

In order to estimate the probability of a disease being inherited it is necessary to appreciate the different patterns of inheritance that can occur.

Autosomal recessive

- Only one generation affected.
- Often onset before adulthood but most recessive diseases include rare cases which are late onset and atypical.
- Commoner in communities with high rates of first cousin marriages (consanguinity).
- Includes most inherited neurological disease due to inborn errors of metabolism (e.g. storage disorders, leucodystrophies).
- Examples: Friedreich's ataxia, Wilson's disease.
- Late onset autosomal recessive disease may be difficult to identify unless the possibility is considered.
- See Figure 6.2 for a typical pedigree.

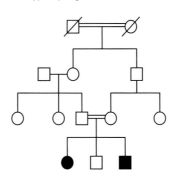

Fig. 6.2 Autosomal recessive pedigree.

Autosomal dominant

- Typically adult onset.
- Age of onset often inversely correlated with severity (early onset more severe).
- Individuals in more that one generation affected.
- If no family history is evident but the phenotype is typical of an autosomal disease (e.g. Huntington's disease) this may indicate:
  - A new mutation.
  - Non-paternity (unknown to the patient).
  - The disease is late onset and family members in previous generations have died of other conditions before reaching the age at which the genetic disease occurs.
  - Variable penetrance: some family members carry the disease causing genetic change but do not manifest the disease due to other modifying genetic factors.

- The family history has been suppressed within the family (not uncommon in diseases like HD).
- The genetic disease was incorrectly diagnosed in other family members. In the pre-MRI era many undiagnosed neurological diseases were labelled as 'multiple sclerosis' and any kind of dementia was usually called 'Alzheimer's disease'.
- See Figure 6.3 for a typical pedigree.

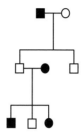

Fig. 6.3 Autosomal dominant pedigree.

Autosomal dominant with reduced penetrance

- The 'penetrance' is defined as the percentage of people who carry the genetic change and manifest the disorder.
- The disease appears to skip a generation because some individuals are protected by other genetic factors or die before they reach the age of onset.
  Fewer individuals are affected than would be expected for autosomal dominant disease.
- Calculating the risk for subsequent family members, even if a gene test is available, is not straightforward.
- See Figure 6.4 for a typical pedigree.

X-linked

  Typically early onset (Kennedy's disease is an exception).
  Males affected only.
- Usually recessive (i.e. females who carry a normal as well as a mutant bearing X-chromosome are not affected).
  Typically affected individuals in one generation only.
  Females can be mildly or subclinically affected (manifesting carriers) due to skewed X-inactivation.
  See Figure 6.5.

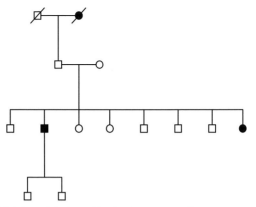

Fig. 6.4 Autosomal dominant with reduced penetrance pedigree.

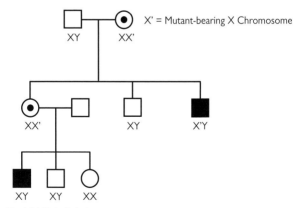

Fig. 6.5 X-linked inheritance.

Mitochondrial

- Most genes that encode protein involved in mitochondrial structure and function are encoded by the nuclear genome, in which case autosomal dominant or recessive inheritance will apply.
- The mitochondrial genome is 16kB in size and encodes genes for components of the respiratory chain, mitochondrial tRNAs, and ribosomal RNA.
- Mitochondrial DNA (mtDNA) from sperm is excluded from the fertilized ovum and thus all mitochondrial DNA is derived from the maternal line.
- Mitochondrial diseases can occur at any age and with variable severity. This is partly explained by heteroplasmy: the load of mutant mtDNA varies between cells and tissues.
- Mutations include missense (e.g. 3243 point mutation leading to MELAS), and mtDNA deletion (leading to progressive external ophthalmoplegia, for instance).
- Susceptible tissues include, liver, muscle, brain, and retina.

Taking a family history

- Between 5 and 10% of patients with typical amyotrophic lateral sclerosis will have a family history of the disease and will thus be classified as having familial ALS.
- Because ALS can also be associated with frontotemporal dementia and also because of the potential importance of neurodegenerative disease clustering in families due to a general 'at risk profile', it is important to take a family history with the appropriate technique (see Box 6.2).
- Bear in mind that family members who died in the distant past without expert neurological evaluation may have been incorrectly labelled as having 'multiple sclerosis' or 'Alzheimer's disease'.

Box 6.2 Guidelines for taking a family history

- Avoid vague or ambiguous questions such as 'does anything run in the family?'
- Ask about each individual in the family, starting with the parents of the affected patient, followed by the siblings. If appropriate ask whether the parents are related. Ways of asking this without causing offence include 'are your parents members of a larger family group?' 'are your parents from the same village or town?'
- If deceased, how old were they when they died? What was the cause of death? What other illnesses did they have?
- If alive, what medical problems do they have?
- Next, ask about grandparents and aunts and uncles.
- Ask about cousins, particularly when consanguinity may be an issue.
- Finally, ask specifically if anyone in the family, near or distant, has a similar problem to the one presented by the patient you are seeing.
- Draw out a full family tree.

Genetic testing and counselling

This is a skilled activity which is best carried out by a trained clinical geneticist or genetics counsellor either in a specialist genetics clinic or a combined neurogenetics clinic. Counselling involves:

- Estimating genetic risk: this is particularly important in diseases with variable penetrance, where the risk cannot simply be stated as 50% for first-degree relatives. It is also relevant in recessive diseases where the recurrence risk depends on the frequency of a particular mutation in a given population.
- Diagnostic testing: where a patient has symptoms and signs of a disease which enable a clinical diagnosis, a genetic test may be confirmatory, and therefore testing of patients in this context is part of a normal diagnostic work-up. However, it should always be remembered that a genetic diagnosis has implications for other family members and the transmission of this information to a family is likely to be performed best in conjunction with genetic services.
- Pre-symptomatic testing: where a relative of a patient with a genetic disease wishes to know their own status. This requires very delicate handling as the implications of such a test, their personal motivation for being tested, and the consequences of a 'bad news' result need to be carefully explored with the individual. This is a skilled consultation which is best performed by trained geneticists and counsellors.
- Pre-natal testing: this requires detailed knowledge of genetics and of the technologies available for diagnosis and testing, and neurologists should therefore refer patients to genetics services.

Familial amyotrophic lateral sclerosis (fALS)

- Between 5 and 10% of patients attending MND clinics give a family history, indicating that MND has occurred in other relatives.
- Given that the incidence of the disease is low (2 per 100,000 population per year), familial occurrence is likely in most cases to indicate a genetically inherited condition rather than the chance association of MND in two members of the same family.
- A family in which the disease appears to skip a generation usually indicates reduced penetrance of a familial form of MND rather than sporadic disease.
- It is important to take a detailed family history in all patients with MND, paying particular attention to any neurological disease and questioning labels like 'MS', Alzheimer's and older terms for MND like 'creeping paralysis' (which often appeared on death certificates).
- The absence of a family history usually allows a confident diagnosis of sporadic ALS to be made, bearing in mind the caveats for autosomal dominant disease (see Patterns of genetic inheritance). Early reassurance that the disease is not likely to be transmitted to children can be very important.
- Whether there is in fact a slightly increased *relative* risk (but still a low *absolute* risk) to first-degree relatives has not yet been determined with certainty.

General clinical characteristics of familial ALS

- Clinically indistinguishable from sporadic disease in individual cases.
- Median age of onset at least 10 years earlier than sALS.
- All subtypes of ALS can be found in the fALS population.
- Penetrance is variable.
- ALS-FTD pedigrees in which the separate phenotypes (ALS, FTD, or ALS-FTD) can occur in isolation or in combination are described.
- For each gene that has been identified (see Table 6.1) as causing fALS mutations have been described in a significant number of patients with 'sporadic ALS'. Although the reasons for this may be complex (new mutations, non-paternity, low penetrance, lack of a reliable family history, and people dying of other causes before reaching the at-risk age), it suggests that mutations in the identified genes may also act as rare risk alleles (in which the presence of a mutation confers a variable and individual risk in conjunction with other genetic and non-genetic factors) as well as clear Mendelian genetic mutations (in which the mutation is the prime determinant of disease). Therefore, the clear separation of sALS and fALS may turn out to be artificial.

Table 6.1 Classification of familial ALS by genetic locus (the shading indicates fALS that cannot be distinguished from sporadic ALS on clinical grounds)

Locus	Gene	Frequency	Clinical
ALS1 (21q22)	SOD1	15-20% of FALS 1-2% of total ALS	Typical ALS
ALS2 (2q33)	Alsin	Rare recessive, mostly in inbred populations	Atypical. Juvenile UMN syndrome resembling PLS
ALS3 (18q21)	Unknown	One family	Typical ALS
ALS4 (9q34)	Senataxin	Very rare	Atypical. Young onset, slow progression, distal weakness with UMN features
ALS5 (15q15)	Unknown	Rare recessive	Atypical. Juvenile onset disease with slow progression
ALS6 (16q12)	FUS	3-5% of FALS	Typical ALS
ALS7 (20p13)	Linkage unconfirmed	One family	Typical ALS
ALS8	VAPB	Very rare, mostly Brazil	Atypical, variable, generally LMN
ALS9 (14q11)	Angiogenin	Rare	Typical ALS
ALS10 (1p36)	TDP-43	1-3% of FALS	Typical ALS
ALS-FTD	9q21/9q21, others	Variable	ALS, FTD, or ALS-FTD

ALS1 due to mutations in the gene for SOD1

- Accounts for <20% of all fALS cases and therefore 2% of all MND patients. It was the first genetic cause of fALS to be identified and has been the subject of intensive research.
- The SOD1 protein is 153 amino acids in length. It is one of the most abundant proteins in the central nervous system. More than 140 mutations have been described in both familial and sporadic ALS (see the ALS genetic database: http://alsod.iop.kcl.ac.uk). Every region of the gene harbours mutations but there is a preponderance in exons 4 and 5.
- All of the mutations cause dominantly inherited fALS with a couple of notable exceptions like the D90A mutation which usually causes recessive inheritance on a Scandinavian genetic background.

- While the penetrance of SOD1 mutations is generally high there are examples of low penetrance alleles, so care must be exercised in counselling about risk to unaffected first-degree relatives.
- There is very little genotype-phenotype correlation in fALS due to SOD1 mutations. Some exceptions are A4V, which causes rapidly progressive disease with death on average within a year, and the D90A recessive mutation, where the disease runs its course typically over 15 years.
- There is a general preponderance of lower motor neuron dominant phenotypes and rapid progression with SOD1 mutations.
- A few mutations are associated with lower-limb onset and slow progression (e.g. H46R, D90A).
- Dementia is very rare.

Pathogenesis
- SOD1 mutations do not lead to disease by a loss of the normal enzyme function in free-radical scavenging
- Mutations lead to misfolded protein which accumulates in motor neurons and glia. Notably, SOD1 cases do not show TDP-43 positive immunostaining.
- A large number of pathways have been implicated in the pathogenesis including mitochondrial dysfunction, neurofilament accumulation, failure of the proteasome, etc. It is not clear which, if any, of these pathways is involved in initiating disease or is secondary to some other pathological process (see Chapter 1).
- Transgenic mouse models (G93A, G85R) have been extensively studied and used to provide evidence for potential therapeutic benefit for many different drugs, none of which to date have shown an effect in human ALS clinical trials.
- Complex transgenic mice in which SOD1 is expressed in a restricted pattern suggest that neurons are the primary cell determining the disease onset, but that glia make a significant contribution to disease expression.

ALS6 due to mutations in the gene for FUS
- FUS ('fused in sarcoma') is an RNA-binding protein which is normally located in the nucleus.
- A number of families with fALS have been identified with mutations, with a predominance in exon 15.
- Autopsy shows accumulation of the protein in cytoplasmic aggregates.
- The disease appears to be clinically indistinguishable from sporadic ALS.
- Mutations have also been identified in sALS patients.

ALS9 due to mutations in the gene for TDP-43
- TAR DNA Binding protein (TDP-43) is the principal protein component of ubiquitinated inclusions which are the pathological hallmark of ALS.
- TDP-43 pathology also occurs in a wide variety of other neurodegenerative diseases, especially in FTD with ubiquitinated inclusions.

- More than 20 mutations across many populations have been identified in ALS patients, both in sporadic and familial disease.
- Mutations cluster in the glycine-rich C-terminal region of the protein, which is thought to bind ribonucleoprotein.
- Clinically the disease is indistinguishable from sporadic ALS.

ALS10 due to mutations in the gene for angiogenin

- Accounts for a small proportion of fALS cases and a very small number of sALS cases.
- Commoner in patients of Irish or Scottish descent.
- Angiogenin is part of a network of proteins involved in tissue response to hypoxia but also has trophic effects on motor neurons in development and in cell culture.

Genetics of sporadic ALS/MND

It is inherently plausible that genetic factors might contribute to the risk of developing sporadic ALS. Any genetic model of sporadic ALS has to provide some explanation for the epidemiological features of ALS described in Chapter 1. Two models are currently proposed:

- **Common variant model**. Candidate gene association studies compare the incidence of variations in a known gene with a putative motor neuron function in cases and controls. Such studies can be criticised because of low sample sizes, failure of replication in subsequent populations, failure to publish negative results, and problems with control groups. The whole genome approach makes no prior assumptions about which genes or loci might be associated with the disease. Several so-called complex diseases (caused by a mixture of genetic and environmental factors) have been analysed using high-throughput genotyping with many hundreds of thousands of markers (usually single nucleotide polymorphisms, SNPs) scattered across the genome. This has revealed that the genetic contribution to Type II diabetes, inflammatory bowel disease, and other conditions consists of multiple (typically 20-30) small effects (relative risk 1.1-1.3) at many genetic loci. This unanticipated level of complexity is likely to increase as we understand more about non-coding genetic variation, copy number variation, and RNA regulation of gene expression. Whole genome studies in ALS so far have not shown a reproducible genetic association at any locus. This indicates that there are no major genetic determinants of ALS with a strong effect that can be observed in mixed populations of ALS patients. However, much larger studies are required to identify or exclude the kind of small effects seen in diabetes and other diseases.
- **Rare variant model.** As mentioned previously in this chapter, it turns out that mutations in Mendelian genes such as SOD1 and TDP-43 occur in patients with sporadic ALS and familial ALS. This can be interpreted as meaning that these rare variations can act as low-penetrance susceptibility alleles. If rare variants in many genes individually explain the genetic contribution for sporadic ALS in a few percent of patients the collective contribution of these variations might be highly significant. As more Mendelian genes are indentified it will become clear if this model is correct.

These two models are not mutually exclusive. It is possible that both make a contribution to genetic risk in individuals, but what is clear is that the genetic contribution to sporadic ALS as a whole is highly complex.

Potential disease-modifying therapies

The history of therapeutic trials in MND

Over 75 compounds have been tried in the treatment of MND without success. Criticisms of clinical trials include:

- Inadequate power:
  - Small numbers of patients.
  - Subject population too heterogeneous (rapid and slow progressors, early and late stage disease patients included together).
- Blunt, insensitive end-points:
  - Survival takes 1–2 years to establish outcome.
  - The ALS Functional Rating Scale is non-linear, may not always reflect disease progression, and may not reflect UMN involvement to the same extent as LMN.
  - Forced vital capacity is insensitive to disease progression until established respiratory involvement, which can occur at any stage of the disease from presentation to terminal phase.
- A lack of biomarkers of disease progression and prognosis. This may improve through:
  - CSF multi-protein profiling.
  - MRI techniques such as diffusion tensor tractography.
  - Better pre-clinical (animal) models.
  - Development of methodology for combination therapies.
- A poor 'translational pipeline':
  - Lack of basic understanding of the disease mechanisms: this is likely to improve with advances in genetics and molecular and cellular biology.
  - Poor *in vitro* drug testing systems: may improve with availability of stem cell models.
  - Too much reliance on evidence of therapeutic benefit in *SOD1* mouse model studies: new models based on TDP-43 mutations may better reflect the pathophysiology of sporadic ALS.

What has been tried?

The most significant drugs used in human clinical trials are listed below:

- Growth factors (rationale: pre-clinical studies indicating neuroprotection):
  - brain-derived neurotrophic factor (BDNF)
  - ciliary neurotrophic factor (CNTF)
  - glial-derived neurotrophic factor (GDNF)
  - insulin-like growth factor (IGF-1).
- Anti-convulsants (rationale: targeting excitotoxicity):
  - gabapentin
  - lamotrigine
  - riluzole
  - topiramate.
- Immuno-modulatory agents (rationale: inhibition of immune response to cellular injury):
  - cyclosporin
  - interferon beta-1a
  - lymphoid irradiation.

- Anti-microbials (various rationales):
  - ceftriaxone (*in vitro* evidence of effects on glutamate transporter editing),
  - indinavir (anti-retroviral; ALS-like syndrome in some HIV cases)
  - minocycline (proposed anti-inflammatory action)
- Anti-inflammatory (rationale: effect on microglial activation):
  - celecoxib.
- Metabolic factors:
  - N-acetylcysteine
  - vitamin E (anti-oxidants)
  - branched-chain amino acids
  - creatine (improved mitochondrial bioenergetics).
- Miscellaneous:
  - arimoclomol (heat shock protein upregulation)
  - buspiron
  - dextromethorphan
  - nimodipine
  - ONO-2506 (inhibition of astrocyte activation)
  - oxandrolone
  - pentoxifylline
  - selegiline (because of effect as neuroprotectant in Parkinson's disease)
  - TCH-346
  - verapamil
  - xaliproden.

Riluzole

Riluzole, a benzothiazole, was originally used in colour photo developing solutions, and initially tested in clinical trials as a potential anti-convulsant due to its broad effect as a glutamate antagonist.

The evidence in ALS
- The first clinical trial results were published in 1994:
- 155 patients, stopped at 21 months:
  - Median survival 544 days using riluzole versus 449 days using placebo.
  - Riluzole reduced mortality by 39% at 12 months (relative risk 0.61; 95% CI 0.39 to 0.97; p=0.014).
- From meta-analyses:
  - ~10% survival benefit. Similar to current chemotherapy for non-small cell carcinoma of the lung.
  - NNT to delay one death at one year is 11.
- National Institute for Clinical Excellence (NICE, the UK body which assesses and approves funding for expensive treatments) approved riluzole in 2001:
  - Panel considered four randomized trials.
  - ~1500 patients.
  - Estimated NHS drug cost ~£3,700 p.a.
  - The drug should only be initiated by a neurological specialist and be prescribed and managed in a cooperative partnership between the hospital specialist and family doctor.

The controversies
There is no clear evidence that in the era in which riluzole has been available the natural history of the disease, as played out in either clinic populations or population registers, has altered. Confounding factors in assessing historical trends in survival include coordinated care, NIV, and PEG, which, if anything, would be expected to contribute to increased survival. Following NICE approval, the decision about whether or not to take the drug should be the patient's informed choice, with the following suggested information having being provided:
- Riluzole is not a cure for MND.
- A clinical trial showed a clear (but only small) survival benefit in the riluzole-treated group.
- Riluzole will not improve symptoms.
- There is no way of knowing the individual patient benefit, which might be greater or less than the overall average benefit in the trial setting.
- Although generally well tolerated, riluzole may make some patients feel worse. In our experience about 10% of people do not tolerate the drug. This is more likely in elderly patients.

Practicalities
- Riluzole is generally a very safe and well-tolerated drug:
- Dose 50mg bd (Rilutek®, Aventis Pharma).
- Riluzole tablets can be crushed and put down a PEG tube.

- Lethargy or nausea are the main reasons why about 10% of patients stop taking the drug.
- Patients should be counseled about the potential effects on driving performance.
- Sustained and significant liver enzyme rises are unusual (2–3% of patients), and the risk of fulminant hepatic failure negligible. A minority of patients have a two- to three-fold elevation in transaminases which plateaus and does not necessarily indicate stopping the drug.
- Neutropenia is also very rare.
- **Contraindications:**
  - hepatic impairment
  - renal impairment
  - neutropenia
  - actual or potential pregnancy
  - breast feeding.
- **Monitoring regime**:
  - baseline bloods (FBC, renal, and LFTs)
  - monthly bloods for first 3 months
  - three-monthly bloods to 1 year
  - annually thereafter.
- Mild elevation of LFTs (<5x upper limit of normal):
  - Halve dose to 50mg od and re-check in 2 weeks.
  - Stop drug if continued rise and check resolution.
- Significant elevation of LFTs (>5x ULN)
  - Stop the drug completely and check resolution.
- Neutropenia requires cessation:
  - Patients should have FBC taken during febrile illnesses.

Non-invasive ventilation

The benefits of non-invasive ventilation are both in symptom control and extending survival (see Chapter 9).

The evidence for improved survival

There is class II and III evidence only (mainly observational studies), using outcome measures of respiratory function (e.g. FVC), survival, and QoL measures:

- 1–2 years survival improvement in positive studies:
  - May reduce chest infections in part.
- May favour those without significant bulbar involvement.
- Variable effects on measures of respiratory function.
- Generally positive effects on symptoms and QoL.

The controversies

- No class I evidence:
  - Ethically/practically challenging to carry out large prospective placebo-controlled trials.
- Publication bias towards studies with positive outcomes.
- Expense of equipment and training.
- Uncertainty about effectiveness in patients with marked bulbar involvement due to secretions.

The potential of stem cells

At present, stem cell therapy for MND represents a long-term aspiration. However, it is a frequent subject of discussion raised by patients and attracts considerable media attention.

What are stem cells?

Stem cells were discovered several decades ago, but it is recent developments in cell separation technology that have allowed their relatively recent manipulation and study. They are defined by two properties:
- Self-renewal – undergo cell division without differentiation.
- Potency – able to differentiate into (usually multiple if pluripotent) specialized cell types.

Where do stem cells come from?

- There are three main sources for stem cells:
- Adult stem cells:
  - Umbilical cord blood (pluripotent).
  - Mesenchymal, endothelial (multipotent within original tissue limits).
  - Used routinely to treat leukaemias through bone marrow transplant.
- Embryonic stem cells:
  - Cells from inner cell mass of embryonic blastocyst (pluripotent).
  - Currently no approved treatment use.
  - Currently requires embryo destruction.
- Induced pluripotent stem cells (iPS):
  - Adult differentiated somatic cells such as skin fibroblasts can be 'reprogrammed' to revert to a multipotent stem cell phenotype using a 'cocktail' of transcription factors delivered by retroviral transduction.
  - Potentially a major advance as there is an infinite and ethically neutral source of cells.
  - At present a very promising tool for research: motor neurons can be derived from somatic cells from patients with familial and sporadic ALS and studied directly in the laboratory.

What are the potential uses in MND?

- Indirectly promote repair or at least arrest pathology:
  - 'Trophic support' to surviving motor neurons to slow disease progression.
  - Increased glial cell numbers.
  - Gene therapy, e.g. stem cells transgenically manipulated to deliver growth factors or other proteins with potential disease-modifying effect.
- Repopulation of motor system and reconstitution of functional pathways:
  - Anterior horn cells and their peripheral motor neurons.
  - Corticospinal tract neurons.
  - Extra-motor cerebral neurons.
  - This is self-evidently a considerably more ambitious aim than simply providing trophic support.

What are the major scientific hurdles?

- A reliable and ethical source of cells:
  - Embryonic stem cells raise many practical and ethical issues.
  - iPS may ultimately provide such as source.
- *Ex-vivo* manipulation:
  - Cells will have to be 'engineered' to produce disease-modifying proteins or to adopt an appropriate motor neuronal phenotype once delivered to the CNS.
- Targeting:
  - Delivery of stem cells to correct location, either directly by implantation (avoiding further damage) or indirectly (systemically with some mechanism for migration to sites of injury). Entry through the blood brain barrier and across vascular endothelium is a major issue to be tackled.
- Viability:
  - Promoting long-term survival of stem cells (e.g. nutrient supply).
  - Preventing host rejection of stem cells.
  - Prevention of disease phenotype affecting transplanted cells.
- Differentiation:
  - CNS environment is 'hard-wired' with specific molecules (e.g. Nogo A) that prevent neuronal outgrowth in the adult.
  - Exact manipulation of stem cells into desired neuronal type will at least in part require differentiation *in situ*.
- Integration:
  - Formation of synapses with existing neurons to reconstitute functional pathways.
- Restriction:
  - Prevention of malignant transformation.
  - Prevention of aberrant synapses.

Further reading

Bensimon G, Lacomblez L, Meininger V (1994). A controlled trial of riluzole in amyotrophic lateral sclerosis. *N Engl J Med*, 330, 585–91.

Miller RG, Mitchell JD, Lyon M, Moore DH (2002). Riluzole for amyotrophic lateral sclerosis (ALS)/motor neuron disease (MND). *Cochrane Database Syst Rev*, 2, CD001447.

Bourke SC, McColl E, Shaw PJ, Gibson GJ (2004). Validation of quality of life instruments in amyotrophic lateral sclerosis. *ALS and other Motor Neuron Disorders*, 5, 55–60.

Symptom management

Muscle symptoms

Spasticity

- Spasticity is a reflection of corticospinal tract (upper motor neuron) damage and has been defined as a 'velocity-dependent increase in muscle tone in response to stretching a relaxed muscle'.
- In the context of MND it is a particular problem in PLS.
- Patients may complain of stiff limbs, difficulty initiating movement, painful spasms, and involuntary movements such as 'jumpiness' of limbs.
- Dyssynergic patterns of co-contraction during movement lead to incoordination and loss of stability.
- It can lead to problems with dexterity, affecting the ability to carry out daily tasks such as personal care, reduced mobility, and increased falls.
- If left untreated it can lead to permanent postural and positioning problems due to secondary contractures.

Management

- Spasticity is best managed by the multidisciplinary team.
- The aim of treatment is to maintain muscle length and range of movement to prevent soft tissue shortening without reducing function.
- Non-pharmacological treatment includes:
  - 24-hour posture and positioning using splints or orthoses.
  - Passive stretching exercises performed by the patient or carer after assessment and advice from a physiotherapist.
- Drug treatment should be considered carefully as it may reduce the stabilizing effect of increased tone and exacerbate the effect of the underlying weakness, e.g. some patients with leg weakness rely on their extensor spasm to stand, transfer, and walk.

Drugs

- Baclofen:
  - GABA agonist.
  - Start at 5–10 mg nocte.
  - Build up slowly, in 5–10 mg increments every 4–5 days, to maximum 30 mg tds.
  - Sedation problematic and doses above 30 mg/day are often not tolerated.
  - Avoid abrupt withdrawal.
  - In rare patients with PLS who are no longer ambulant, intrathecal baclofen delivered via a programmable infusion pump directly into the CSF is an option to consider. It is expensive and requires a specialist unit for insertion and to supervise management. The small doses of baclofen required to block GABA receptors locally in the spinal cord effectively eliminate systemic unwanted effects such as drowsiness.
- Tizanidine:
  - Alternative to baclofen.
  - Start at 2 mg nocte.
  - Build up in 2 mg increments every 3–4 days to maximum 8–12 mg tds.
  - Needs LFT check at baseline and with increases until stable.
  - Sedation can be problematic.

- Dantrolene:
  - Alternative to baclofen and tizanidine but rarely used due to frequent unwanted effects (including sedation).
  - Start at 25 mg daily.
  - Increased in 25 mg increments weekly to maximum 75–100 mg tds.
- Gabapentin:
  - GABA analogue.
  - Useful for treating painful spasms.
  - Dose should be increased and decreased gradually.
  - Start at 300 mg od and build up to 600 mg tds over several weeks.
  - Some patients cannot tolerate high doses due to drowsiness.
- Benzodiazepines:
  - Effective for acute relief of exacerbations of spasticity.
  - Tolerance develops, with potential for dependence.
  - Can exacerbate respiratory insufficiency.
  - Diazepam 2.5–5 mg up to qds or clonazepam 0.5–2 mg up to qds.
- Botulinum toxin:
  - Potent neurotoxin injected into specific target muscles.
  - Temporarily uncouples nerve from muscle at the neuromuscular junction by preventing the release of acetylcholine from the pre-synaptic nerve terminal.
  - Used cautiously in patients with MND as it results in reduced muscle contraction and muscle power.
  - Effect is temporary, lasting up to 3–4 months and then needs repeating.
  - Generally reserved for patients who cannot walk.

Cramps

- Sudden tightening of individual muscles that can be sustained and leave residual pain:
  - also reflects corticospinal tract (UMN) involvement
  - activated by movement, especially stretching
  - overlap with spasticity.
- Often worse at night.
- Exacerbating factors:
  - cold
  - anxiety
  - caffeine
  - some drugs, e.g. asthma inhalers.
- Prominent in early disease but often fade with progression in ALS.
  - May be persistent in PLS.
- Involve a Physiotherapist early in assessment; massage can be effective in both treating and preventing cramps.

Drugs

- See Spasticity.
- in addition there is limited evidence to support the use of quinine sulphate 200–300 mg at night for cramps in MND.

Fasciculations
- Irregular, chaotic twitching of muscle fibres:
  - Can occur as a normal phenomenon in healthy people (especially after exercise).
  - The origin of fasciculations is still debated. In MND fasciculations reflect anterior horn cell death (LMN) – the surviving neurons at the junction with the muscle make poor additional connections (partial re-innervation) to compensate for the denervation elsewhere. This makes the motor unit electrically unstable. There may also be a contribution from axonal hyperexcitability and also from dysregulation of local spinal cord circuits.
- Prominent in early disease but generally fade with progression:
  - Only rarely are they the patient's presenting symptom.
  - Rarely intrusive enough to require treatment.
  - No clear relationship clinically between frequency and disease severity or progression.
- Exacerbating factors:
  - caffeine
  - alcohol
  - temperature changes.

Drugs
- Beta blockers:
  - propranolol 40 mg od-tds
  - atenolol 25–50 mg od
  - contraindicated in asthma and some cardiac conditions.
- Baclofen (see Spasticity).

Bulbar symptoms

At least 80% of all MND patients (more with PLS) will develop symptomatic speech and swallowing dysfunction (i.e. damage to corticobulbar tract UMNs or cranial nerve LMNs IX, X, XII). Although greatly feared by patients, who anticipate becoming 'locked in' and unable to express their feelings or wishes, it is not a universal or inevitable feature of the disease. Furthermore, many patients with bulbar symptoms retain the ability to communicate with assistance throughout the course of their illness. However, for those affected, bulbar symptoms are a major source of distress.

The management of nutrition, including dysphagia, in MND is covered in detail in Chapter 10.

Sialorrhoea

- A common and troublesome problem in those with bulbar disease. Difficult to treat. Most evidence is from open-label studies with low numbers in treatment group.
- Both sympathetic (increases thick protein-rich secretion) and parasympathetic (increases serous component) activity contribute to saliva production.
- Not primarily an increase in production of saliva, but a failure to clear effectively:
  - Drooling and pooling result.
  - Socially disabling.
  - Can lead to choking attacks and discomfort lying flat.
  - Can prevent or hinder NIV use.
  - Exacerbated by head drop due to neck weakness. Improving head support may help.
- Reducing thick secretions:
  - Avoid dehydration and excessive dairy products.
  - Boiled sweets may help but avoid if aspiration a risk.
  - Pineapple or papaya juice contain lytic enzymes which may help dissolve secretions.
  - Steam inhalation may help.
  - Consider mucolytic drugs e.g. carbocisteine 125–500 mg qds (rarely can cause peptic ulceration); available as liquid (125 mg/mL).
  - There is limited evidence that beta blockers may reduce the thickness of secretions.
- Reducing thin secretions:
  - Requires drug therapy (see below).
  - Balanced approach to avoid rendering the secretions too thick and tenacious as a result.

Drugs

- Hyoscine (scopolamine) hydrobromide
  - 1 mg patch behind ear changed every 3 days.
  - Can cause drowsiness, confusion in the elderly, blurred vision, and urinary hesitancy.
  - Avoid in glaucoma.
  - Two patches can be tried simultaneously if required and otherwise tolerated.

- Amitriptyline:
  - Start at 10 mg nocte.
  - Build up in 10 mg increments weekly to maximum of 100 mg/day. However, doses above 50 mg often cause unacceptable side effects.
  - Also helpful for emotional lability.
  - Can reduce nocturia (but may cause retention).
  - Avoid in glaucoma and in those at risk of urinary retention.
  - Avoid abrupt withdrawal at higher doses.
- Atropine sulphate:
  - 1% eye drops; off-license indication.
  - Two drops sublingually 2–3 times per day. Effect lasts for several hours and can be particularly helpful for controlling saliva for short periods at times to suit the individual.
  - Systemic effects of atropine rare, but possible with overuse and in elderly.
- Ipratropium bromide:
  - Delivered via inhaler pump under the tongue.
  - Small studies have been carried out in Parkinson's disease, showing limited effectiveness.
- Glycopyrronium bromide (glycopyrrolate):
  - Anti-muscarinic structurally related to atropine but longer acting and does not cross the blood-brain barrier.
  - Tablets 1 or 2 mg, start at 0.5 mg orally, one to three times daily; titrate to effectiveness and tolerability.
  - Oral formulation not always easily available in the UK, so can be given intramuscularly or subcutaneously; 200 micrograms IM up to qds.
- Botulinum toxin:
  - Works by chemodenervation at parasympathetic neurosecretory synapses.
  - Judicious peri-salivary gland (parotid/submandibular) injections can be helpful.
  - Success is operator dependent. EMG or ultrasound guidance increases likelihood of beneficial effect.
  - Potential side effects include dysphagia and increased risk of aspiration.
  - Effect wears off and needs repeating every 2–3 months.

Radiotherapy

Radiotherapy to the salivary glands is supported by anecdotal evidence of good effect. There is a potential for problems with dental caries and mucosal breakdown, but these have not been extensively reported. Given the range of other available options this is probably a treatment reserved for exceptional circumstances.

Dry mouth

Causes:
- jaw closure weakness leading to mouth breathing, especially during sleep.
- overuse of measures to address drooling.
- inappropriate use of oxygen.

- Treatment:
  - ice cubes
  - Biotene™ (mouthwash, toothpaste, or gel)
  - artificial saliva sprays (e.g. Glandosane™)
  - saline nebulizers (but avoiding oxygen).

Dysphagia
- See Chapter 10.

Dysarthria
- Eight times more common than dysphagia as a presenting symptom of MND.
- Affects 80% of limb-onset patients at some point in the course of disease; effective residual communication is still possible in many.
- Usually a combination of stiffness (UMN, associated with brisk jaw jerk and other facial reflexes) or floppiness (LMN, associated with tongue wasting) involving:
  - tongue
  - palate
  - jaw
  - larynx.
- Where upper motor neuron features predominate, the characteristic pattern is of spastic dysphonia with slow, strained speech with nasal and oral escape ('hot potato speech').
- Some patients have relatively clear speech but major weakness of vocal cord adduction leading to hypophonia and whispering speech.
- Abnormalities of respiratory function contribute to dysarthria:
  - Production of normal volume sounds requires an adequate vital capacity.
  - Dyskinetic breathing leads to lack of coordination with speech.
- 'Ambulant anarthrics':
  - Patients who become rapidly unable to speak but retain good limb strength for many months afterwards.
- Major source of social isolation and handicap.
- Role of Speech & Language Therapist: assessment, teaching methods to improve intelligibility:
  - slowing the speech rate
  - speaking face to face
  - substituting articulation manoeuvres such as alternative words, spelling, repetition, overarticulating consonants, or even using key words or monosyllabic speech.
- Palatal lift and augmentation prostheses have been tried in patients with a weak palate but usually produce no useful effect due to progression of the disease process, and are therefore not recommended.
- Augmentative and alternative communication aids:
  - Success with complex solutions to communication loss requires specialist input, patience on the part of therapist and patient, and is most likely to benefit patients with slowly progressive MND and prolonged survival.
  - Portable microphone systems for hypophonia.
  - Wipe-clean pen pads (require reasonable hand function).

- Speech synthesis software for use on laptops.
- Voice synthesizers such as the Lightwriter™ device require reasonable hand function. Enables the operator to type in words which will be displayed in visual form or as synthesized speech. The Lightwriter™ can be adapted to individual requirements. If typing separate letters becomes difficult the switches can be changed. The switch can be adapted so that it can be triggered by any part of the body including head, foot, and elbow.
- Ideally patients should learn to use these aids before communication is completely lost. In our experience patients who are able to write will rarely engage in using a Lightwriter™ but continue to use pen and paper as it is considered to be less stigmatizing.
- 'Voice banking' systems exist in which the patient's own characteristic vocal sound is digitized and incorporated into voice synthesis software. This is still developing and currently requires many hours of data banking while the patient is in the early stages of the illness, making it an impractical option for all but the most motivated.
- Travellers' 'Point It'™ books (Graf editions).
- Pointing board with the alphabet, common phrases or pictures.
- Email and mobile phone texting are recent innovations that have dramatically improved communication for MND patients and have reduced social isolation.
- Eye-tracking software can be used to control a computer cursor to drive a voice-synthesizer program. Given the significant period of training required these are most suitable for patients who have slowly progressive disease.

Emotionality

Very common accompaniment to those with corticobulbar involvement.

Has many synonyms: emotional 'lability' or 'incontinence', 'pathological laughter and crying', 'involuntary emotional expression disorder', 'pseudobulbar affect'.

Reduced control over response to emotional stimuli:
- Inappropriate or more easily triggered crying (more rarely laughing too).
- Laughing may turn into crying.
- Difficult to suppress once 'trigger' pulled.

Due to involvement of the corticobulbar pathways:
- Best considered as an abnormal motor response with failure to suppress reflex crying and laughing.
- Although it occurs with a higher frequency in patients with cognitive involvement, it can occur in people with normal cognition.
- It is important to reassure patients, relatives, and other health care professionals that it is not a sign of more widespread cognitive impairment *per se*.

Can be very socially disabling and send 'wrong signals' about mood to others.

- Not infrequently a transient feature of MND and does not progress in tempo with other motor aspects of the disease.
- Many patients are satisfied with a reassuring explanation and do not require drug treatment.

Drugs
- Amitriptyline:
  - Start at 10 mg nocte.
  - Build up in 10 mg increments weekly to maximum of 100 mg.
  - 'Hangover' morning sedation can be problematic (avoid in glaucoma and in those at risk of urinary retention).
  - Avoid abrupt withdrawal.
- SSRIs may also be beneficial (e.g. fluvoxamine).
- A randomized controlled trial of the combination of dextromethorphan and quinidine (the latter inhibits the first pass metabolism of the former) showed benefit but the drug combination (Neurodex, Avanir Pharmaceuticals) is not currently licensed in the UK.

Jaw clenching
- Reflects UMN involvement and failure of reflex inhibitory suppression of the masseter.
- In combination with a stiff tongue, can result in painful biting of tongue.

Drugs
- See Spasticity.

Excessive yawning
- Frequently observed in patients with corticobulbar involvement.
- May reflect more diffuse brainstem involvement.
- Generally hard to treat but can trigger painful jaw spasms (see above) and occasionally causes temperomandibular joint dysfunction or even dislocation.

Increased coughing
- Failure of suppression of the cough reflex.
- Can be treated with cough suppressants such as codeine or dextromethorphan but caution is required to prevent respiratory suppression and increased risk of aspiration.

Laryngeal spasm
- A particularly distressing acute symptom defined as the sudden sensation of the inability to breathe.
- Accompanied by stridor.
- Arises through adduction of the laryngeal muscles and usually lasts for <30 seconds.
- May occur during attempted intubation.
- Can be precipitated by occult or symptomatic gastro-oesophageal reflux which should be treated with proton-pump inhibitors and postural adjustment to reduce the frequency of attacks.

Acute management:
- Calm reassurance that the episode will pass.
- Bracing of the arms and trunk.
- Frequent clusters can be terminated with sub-lingual lorazepam (0.5 mg).

Sleep disturbance

Sleep fragmentation can be an early sign of impending respiratory insufficiency (see Chapter 9).

Important to consider non-respiratory causes of frequent waking:
- General immobility leading to difficulty in turning in bed.
- Joint pains; can be treated by nightly analgesia such as paracetamol.
- Mood disturbance, ranging from temporary psychological adjustment reactions to frank depression.
- Anxiety or panic attacks.
- Coughing; can be treated with postural adjustments and cough suppressants.

Bowel and bladder management

Sphincter disturbance as a direct result of pathological involvement in MND is very unusual, but secondary involvement due to immobility is common, and can cause significant erosion of quality of life.

Constipation

- Causes:
  - Immobility and lack of exercise.
  - Weakness of pelvic floor muscles.
  - Dehydration.
  - A change to a softer diet when dysphagia occurs leads to a reduction in fibre intake.
  - Rarely, autonomic involvement in the disease process may be a factor.
  - Drugs: opioid analgesics.
  - Psychological factors: dependence on others for help, immobility, etc.
- Dietary management: advice from a dietitian about increasing fibre (e.g. high-fibre cereals softened with milk, bananas, etc.).
- Establishment of a good 'bowel routine' with dedicated time allocated after breakfast when the gastrocolic reflex is at its height.

Drugs

- Lactulose:
  - Osmotic laxative that relies on a good oral fluid intake, and so rarely effective in established constipation.
  - 15 mL bd.
- Senna:
  - 2–4 tablets taken nocte.
- Docusate:
  - Up to 500 mg in divided doses per day (available as liquid).
- Movicol:
  - Very helpful in acute setting and to establish a regular pattern.
  - 1–3 sachets dissolved in water, divided over day.
  - Higher doses can be used for acute faecal disimpaction.

Urinary urgency

- MND patients with UMN-predominant disease can experience mild urinary urgency.
- Very common in PLS.
- Nocturia disturbs sleep and increases the risk of falls.
- A sheath with leg bag can be helpful in men, especially overnight, though often causes difficulties with sheath retention.
- 'Convenience' invasive catheterization is best avoided due to complications of infection but may be justified in patients with a high level of dependency, in which case a suprapubic catheter is often the best option.

Drugs

Amitriptyline:
- Used for its anti-cholinergic side effects which promote bladder retention, but sedative properties can also be useful at night unless there is overt respiratory insufficiency.
- Start at 10 mg nocte.
- Build up in 10 mg increments weekly to maximum of 100 mg.
- 'Hangover' morning sedation can be problematic (avoid in glaucoma).
- Avoid abrupt withdrawal at higher doses.

Alternative anti-cholinergics:
- oxybutynin 2.5–5 mg nocte–bd
- tolterodine 1–2 mg bd.

Acid indigestion

Dyspepsia is a common complaint in the older age group but is exacerbated by prolonged recumbency and 'stress' in MND.

Weakness of the diaphragm contributes to incompetence of the oesophageal sphincter.

May be a precipitant of laryngospasm.

NSAIDs may be required for joint pain and these will exacerbate or promote acid indigestion (and even peptic ulceration).

Gastritis, duodenitis, or peptic ulceration may be found during PEG insertion, and may require formal *H. pylori* eradication therapy.

Antacids are generally best given at night when acid production is maximal.

Drugs

Gaviscon:
- 5–10 mL after meals and nocte.

Ranitidine:
- 150 mg nocte-bd.

Proton-pump inhibitor, e.g. omeprazole 20–40 mg nocte.

Pro-kinetic agents:
- especially with PEG *in situ*
- domperidone 10–20 mg tds-qds.

Symptoms related to immobility

Joint pain
- Pain arising in MND is most commonly mechanical pain arising from joints.
- Loss of peri-articular muscle tone leads to joint instability, especially of the shoulder and hip.
- Pre-existing low back pain is greatly exacerbated by immobility.
- Inability to turn in a chair or bed to adequately relieve discomfort makes symptoms difficult to tolerate and disturbs sleep.
- Regular analgesia is more likely to be beneficial, rather than reacting when pain is at its peak.
- Specific advice from a specialist physiotherapist to assess posture and support of specific joints with slings, braces, and neck collars.
- Assessment for a specialist profiling bed with electronic controls to adjust posture.

Drugs
- Paracetamol:
  - 1 g max 6-hourly qds.
- Non-selective NSAIDs carry risk of peptic ulceration with prolonged use, and are best combined with an anti-acid drug (see Acid indigestion):
  - ibuprofen 200–400 mg tds
  - naproxen 250–500 mg bd
  - diclofenac SR 75 mg nocte (helpful for overnight cover).
- Selective COX-2 inhibitors have a better GI profile but carry some concerns about long-term cardiovascular safety:
  - E.g. celecoxib 100–200 mg nocte-bd.
- Opiate-containing analgesics are best avoided due to constipating effects and adverse effects on breathing.

Dependent oedema & pressure sores
- Prolonged immobility of the lower limbs frequently results in distal oedema due to raised venous pressure from loss of muscle tone and alterations in neurogenic mechanisms for vasomotor regulation, resulting in:
  - poor skin perfusion and discolouration
  - increased risk of skin breakdown and pressure sore formation
  - increased risk of venous thrombosis.
- Compression stockings can be helpful but inconvenient to wear.
- Keeping lower limbs raised slightly when seated or raising the foot end of the bed by 10 cm may help.
- Diuretics are best avoided as they promote urinary urgency and electrolyte disturbance.
- Although MND patients are in principle a high-risk group for pressure sores, it is a relatively rare problem.

- Emphasis is on prevention:
  - Attention to dependent skin areas and early recognition of 'at risk' erythema.
  - Attention to overnight turning where patient can no longer initiate.
  - Turning problems may be relieved by 'sliding sheets'.
  - Speedy provision of appropriate hospital air-compressed mattress when indicated.
- Established pressure sores require aggressive monitoring and treatment.

Psychological & psychiatric symptoms

Risk of suicide (see also Chapter 2)

- The approach to conveying the diagnosis of MND outlined in Chapter 2 minimizes the possibility of a catastrophic psychological reaction.
- However, there are some individuals who require immediate extra support and there are rare instances of attempted suicide in this context.
- There was a 5–6 fold overall increase in suicide in ALS patients compared to the background population in one Swedish study.
- Identifying patients at risk is not straightforward, but suicide is more likely in the first year of the disease, in younger patients, in those living alone, and in people with a previous psychiatric history.

Depression

- There is an ongoing debate as to whether clinically significant depression appears neither as prevalent nor as severe as might be expected, given the nature of MND, or whether it is just underdiagnosed.
- Subclinical dysexecutive function could confound the assessment of depressive symptoms.
- MND patients are more likely to suffer a sense of hopelessness.
- Carers are at high risk of depression, especially for patients on invasive ventilation.
- In the patient, depression can have secondary effects on calorific intake and mobility, as well as influencing suicidal ideation.
- A simple tool to assess depression in the clinic is the Beck Depression Inventory.

Drugs

- SSRIs:
  - E.g. sertraline 50 mg daily.
  - May be used in conjunction with amitriptyline but can increase the plasma concentration.
- NB St John's Wort is a complementary therapy that can adversely interact with other prescribed medications including SSRIs.

Cognitive impairment (see also Chapter 3)

- Mild dysexecutive syndrome is common in MND, but rarely clinically apparent and unlikely to represent a 'capacity' issue.
- Frank dementia is rare (<5%):
  - Frontotemporal in nature (FTD).
  - FTD can precede the onset of MND (especially primary progressive aphasic form).
  - Usually associated with faster progression of motor disease.
- Clinical features generally 'negative' rather than 'positive':
  - Personality change or blunting.
  - Apathy.
  - Little or no insight.
  - May be well preserved procedural memory, e.g. driving.

- Altered food preference, often narrowed and favouring sweet foods.
  - Food cramming (can precipitate choking).
  - Disinhibition (usually verbal but can extend to physical neglect).
- Initial management includes the exclusion of other conditions which can confound or mimic cognitive impairment:
  - Depression.
  - Severe withdrawal as an adjustment reaction to diagnosis.
  - Hypoxia from respiratory involvement.
  - Drugs.
  - Other coexisting illness (e.g. hypothyroidism).
- The presence of cognitive decline has major implications for engaging patients in interventions such as PEG.
- Involve extended family members early where there are concerns about capacity or vulnerabilities arising from lack of self-care.
- Severe behavioural disturbance as part of MND-FTD is unusual:
  - Seek advice of Old Age Psychiatrist and Neuropsychologist.
  - Consider atypical neuroleptics e.g. quetiapine and risperidone.

Complementary therapies

Loosely defined as treatments outside the realm of 'conventional' medical practice. Many patients report improvements in well-being with massage, acupuncture, and other therapies for which there is no established evidence base. One study suggested 50% of MND patients use complementary therapies, with significant financial outlay in many cases. The distinction between 'conventional' versus 'alternative' is not helpful. Another way of viewing treatment is in the following categories:

- Treatments that are effective.
- Treatments that are ineffective.
- Treatments that are harmful, including:
  - Adverse interactions with other therapies.
  - Financial harm if they are expensive.
  - Psychological harm if they provide false hope.

Effective and ineffective treatments can each be harmful.

Commonly discussed therapies

- No evidence of benefit or harm:
  - Acupuncture.
  - Massage.
  - Reflexology.
  - Homeopathy.
- No evidence of benefit and potentially harmful:
  - Current stem cell therapies.
  - Chelation therapy.
  - Exclusion diets.
  - Certain herbal remedies, chemicals, powders, extracts.
  - Removal of dental fillings.
  - Urine therapy.

A suggested approach

- Non-confrontational, non-judgmental:
  - Better to know about all treatments a patient is taking or considering.
  - Informs understanding of patient's health and illness beliefs.
  - Inappropriate to apply standards of evidence to spiritual belief systems.
  - Use of complementary therapies may be surrogate marker for better outcome due to generally greater motivation.
- Remind patients that many 'mainstream' drugs are also plant-derived and so 'natural'.

Further reading

Oliver D, Walsh D, Borasio GD (2000). *Palliative Care in Amyotrophic Lateral Sclerosis.* Oxford University Press, Oxford.

Management of respiratory symptoms

Assessment of respiratory symptoms

The inevitable development of respiratory muscle (diaphragmatic and intercostal) weakness is the main mechanism leading to premature death in MND. In about 2% of cases, respiratory weakness is the presenting feature, but even in this setting it is usually insidious and can be difficult to recognize in the early stages. Identification of respiratory insufficiency is a key area of management in MND:

- Many symptoms are amenable to treatment.
- Prevention and early management of infection is important.
- Maintenance of well-being through promotion of restorative sleep.
- Reduction of anxiety.

The nature of respiratory involvement in MND

Respiratory involvement in MND is often considered rather narrowly as simply a matter of lower motor neuron weakness of the intercostal muscles, the diaphragm, and ultimately the accessory muscles of breathing. However, as with any other aspect of motor function there are more complex levels of nervous system control and organization which must be considered to gain a full appreciation of the evolution of respiratory symptomatology:

- Voluntary initiation or inhibition of breathing arising in the cortex.
- Corticobulbar and bulbar pathways:
  - Extramotor regulation of arousal and awareness in the cerebral cortex, hypothalamus, amygdala, and periaqueductal grey matter of the midbrain control respiration during speech, locomotion, and response to stress.
  - Similarly, swallowing, coughing, and sneezing require integration with breathing and dysregulation of these reflexes may contribute to the risk of aspiration.
  - Patients with significant corticobulbar involvement, especially those with PLS, may not be able to coordinate a breath during measurement of FVC, which may give a falsely low reading. The same problem can interfere with sniff-nasal pressure measurements (see Sniff-nasal pressure).
- Respiratory pattern generating networks in the brainstem:
  - Control of respiratory rhythm depends on specialized groups of neurons in the pons and medulla which, in the absence of voluntary control such as in 'locked-in' patients, generate a regular breathing rate of 16 breaths per minute. In experimental animals damage to a group of neurons in the ventral medulla known as the pre-Botzinger complex causes the respiratory rhythm to cease.
  - These neurons are in synaptic contact with other local networks which are sensitive to changes in pH and CO_2 and can be overridden by voluntary control of breathing.
  - We are not aware of a pathological study that demonstrates that these neurons are involved in MND but in a minority of patients there appears to be a loss of the involuntary components of breathing control. This is often manifest as an acute awareness of the need to breathe and clinically is easy to mistake for hyperventilation due to anxiety. Notably, such patients will appear

normal by all conventional respiratory tests, though may have abnormal overnight oximetry.
- However, there is a high risk of sudden death, usually within sleep, and these patients are extremely sensitive to low dose benzodiazepines and opioids, which can cause respiratory arrest.
- Spinal pathways provide the final common pathway for movement:
  - Coordinated breathing requires integration of local spinal circuits and bilateral activation of the diaphragm via the phrenic nerve.
  - The diaphragm contributes 2/3 of vital capacity.
  - Asymmetrical lower motor neuron degeneration may lead to dysconjugate breathing, and coupled with postural muscle weakness may require adjustments to seating and beds.
  - Expiration is mostly by elastic recoil of the chest wall and lungs and therefore MND preferentially affects inspiration.

History

The following symptom inquiry list is a good screen for respiratory involvement in MND:

- Are you breathless: (a) at rest; (b) on minimal exertion; (c) on significant exertion; (d) bending over?
- Are you able to lie flat comfortably?
- Do you sleep well at night? If not, why not?
- Have you recently been waking at night to pass water?
- Have you recently changed your sleeping pattern, e.g. prefer to lie on one side?
- Do you wake refreshed in the morning?
- Have you noticed that you have lost your appetite for breakfast recently?
- Do you have early morning nausea or headache?
- Do you have difficulty avoiding dropping off to sleep when you do not choose to while: (a) reading quietly in a chair; (b) as a passenger in a car; (c) at any other time?

Overt breathlessness is not the commonest or earliest symptom of respiratory muscle involvement in MND. The relationship between measurements of respiratory muscle strength such as FVC (see Forced vital capacity) and symptoms of respiratory failure is not an exact one in MND and is determined by factors such as the speed of decline and the pattern of muscle weakness, as well as the relative contributions of the different central regulators of breathing discussed previously. This is an area in which further research is needed. However, it is clear that for a given level of FVC there is a wide range of possible symptoms. It is even possible for patients to progress to terminal respiratory failure without ever feeling breathless.

Physical examination

- The patient should be observed during quiet breathing for:
  - Respiratory rate (normal 12–16 breaths per minute).
  - Ability to talk in full sentences. Patients with significant corticobulbar dysarthria may have significant difficulty speaking but it is still possible to assess respiratory reserve by paying attention to the pattern of breathing during speech.

- Use of accessory muscles of respiration, namely sternomastoid, platysma, shoulders (voluntary shoulder lifting is a particular feature which should alert the observer to the presence of severe respiratory muscle weakness).
- Typical features of lung disease such as cyanosis are not likely to occur in MND patients except immediately pre-mortem.
- Examination of the chest where indicated to exclude infection or other pathology which could compromise breathing.
- Specific assessment of the diaphragm can be made by observing breathing with the patient lying flat. Normally the abdominal wall expands outwards during inspiration. When the diaphragm is weak the abdominal wall contracts inwards. This time-honoured method of observing 'paradox' does not always add much to the examination of the patient with MND, where measurement of FVC lying and sitting is an essential part of the clinical assessment.

Forced vital capacity

This provides the most portable and practical method of monitoring the onset and progression of respiratory involvement in MND. For the majority of patients it is a technically feasible and reliable measure with good inter-rater reliability. There is a wealth of experience from clinical trials to support FVC as a reliable indicator of disease progression. However, for the reasons outlined previously, patients with significant upper or lower motor neuron bulbar involvement may not be easy to assess reliably.

- Portable and reasonably priced desktop spirometers are ideal for the MND clinic. To avoid having to attend a separate appointment this should be available for use by the clinic team, who will rapidly become expert in its use.
- The most helpful way to express FVC is as a percentage of predicted, based on height, gender, etc. Desktop spirometers are programmed in this way.
- We routinely use a mask, rather than a mouthpiece, for all patients.
- Technique is important. The patient should be instructed about creating a seal around their mouth and that all of the air must be expelled in one breath. Three attempts should be made, taking the best effort as a measure of FVC.
- At each clinic visit a lying and sitting measurement should be made, although this may present challenges for patients who are confined to a wheelchair. A tilt-in-space electric chair can facilitate lying FVC measurements. Cautious improvisation, with an assistant tilting back a manual wheelchair, taking necessary precautions to support the patient, can also be useful.
- Interestingly, respiratory symptoms can first occur over a variable range of predicted FVC, from 80% to 40%.
- Diaphragm weakness is suggested by a >20% fall in FVC on lying flat.

Sniff-nasal pressure

In patients in whom measuring FVC is technically unsatisfactory, measurement of SNP is worth trying. It measures the pressure produced at the nose during a maximum inspiratory sniff and requires specialist equipment similar in size and cost to a desktop spirometer. This will not be available in routine outpatient settings and has to be purchased specially. An SNP greater than 40 cmH$_2$O suggests adequate respiratory function.

Overnight oximetry

- The differential diagnosis of sleep disturbance is wide (see p. 127) and therefore objective measures of respiratory function during sleep are very valuable.
- Unexpected abnormalities can be revealed in patients with apparently unexplained symptoms who appear to have reasonable function as measured by clinic FVC.
- We have therefore developed a low threshold for performing overnight oximetry in any patient who appears to have disrupted sleep without an adequate explanation.
- The equipment can be posted out to the patients with instructions for use and does not require an overnight hospital admission.
- Some examples of abnormal patterns are shown in Figure 9.1.

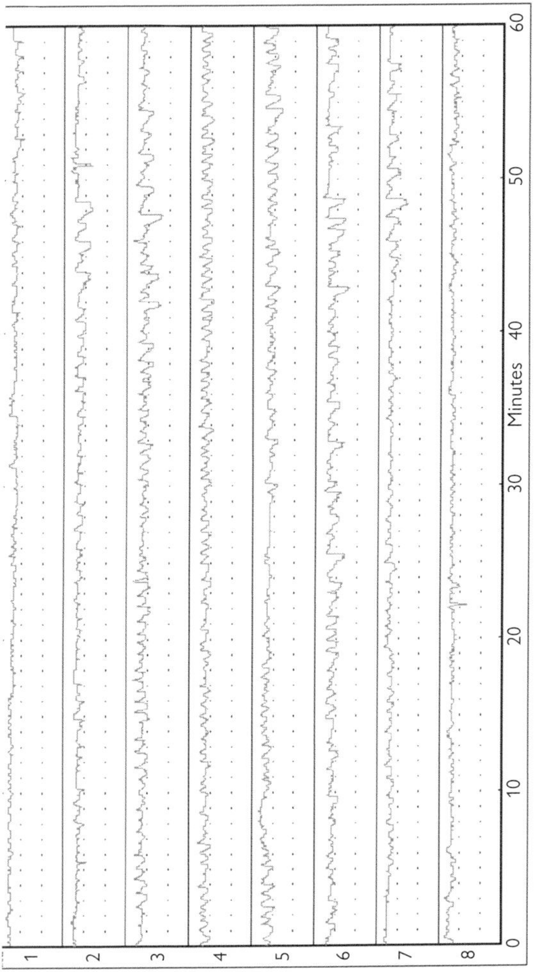

Fig. 9.1a Overnight oximetry from an MND patient who is not yet in ventilatory failure (resting SaO2 at beginning normal). There are no large REM related dips. His predominant pattern is recurrent dips throughout the night, drops in SaO2 with arousal and rapid response.

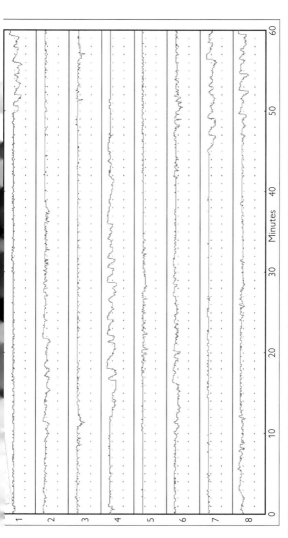

Fig. 9.1b This patient is already in diurnal failure (note low starting SaO2) and there are extra dips during REM.

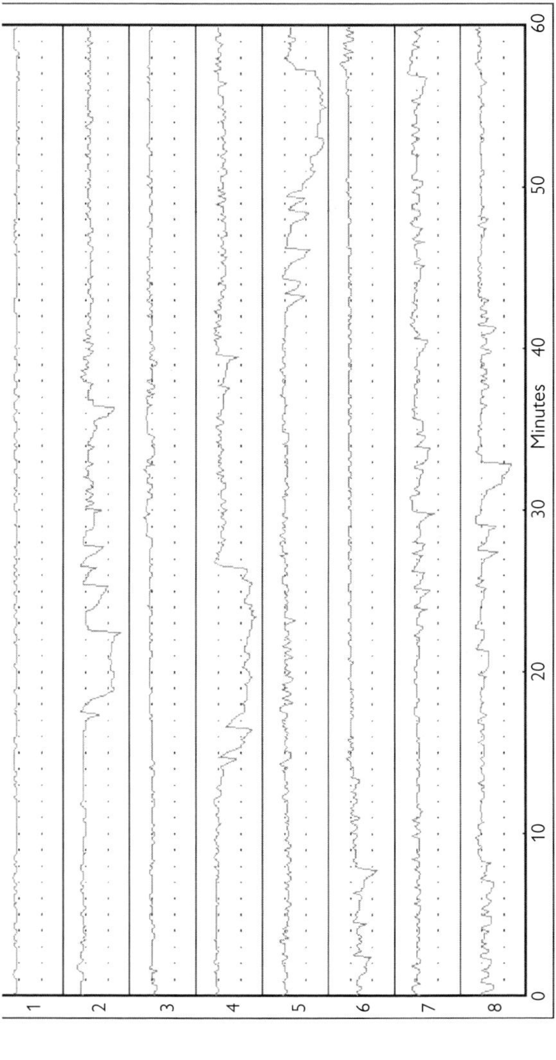

Fig. 9.1c In this patient the RFM dips are bigger suggesting a major diaphragmatic component.

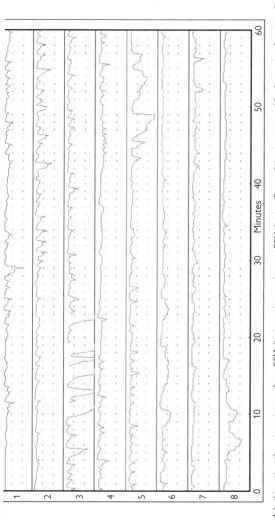

Fig. 9.1d In this patient there is a mixture of non-REM dipping and more dramatic REM dipping (Figures 9.1a–d courtesy of Professor John Stradling, Churchill Hospital, Oxford).

Blood tests

- Routine biochemistry can reveal a low chloride level, which should raise the suspicion of a high bicarbonate (i.e. a partially corrected respiratory acidosis) and prompt further investigation with blood gases.
- The earliest abnormality reliably detected on arterial blood gas analysis is a raised bicarbonate level reflecting renal compensation and a degree of chronicity of hypoventilation. This should be performed in the morning; pCO_2 can be normal at this point with the patient sitting up and alert.
- Hypercapnia during the day occurs as weakness progresses.
- Significantly raised pCO_2 indicates a poor prognosis unless mechanical ventilation is instituted.
- If there is significant hypoxia with normocapnia, it is unlikely to be due to neuromuscular weakness and another cause should be sought.

Specific symptoms

Dyspnoea

- Exercise intolerance due to dyspnoea may be an early warning of respiratory weakness, but MND patients will fatigue more easily anyway due to the generalized effect of muscle weakness on performance.
- Unprovoked 'air hunger' (gasping for air, especially at night), may be a sign of significant respiratory muscle weakness but must be distinguished from 'panic attacks'.
- Always consider co-morbidities that might produce or exacerbate MND-related dyspnoea, e.g. cardiac insufficiency or pulmonary embolism. Sudden development of breathlessness is unusual in MND and should provoke a careful search for a reversible cause.
- MND patients, through immobility, are at high risk for pulmonary embolism:
  - Sudden-onset dyspnoea, pleuritic chest pain, cyanosis, or tachycardia.
  - There is often no clinically obvious lower-limb DVT, though it may be discovered on ultrasound.
  - The slow development of peripheral cyanosis might indicate the accumulation of pulmonary micro-emboli.
  - The use of prophylactic heparin injections or low-dose warfarin to prevent PEs is not generally recommended in palliative care. However, it may be appropriate in individual cases where PE is a feature at earlier stages in the disease.
  - Non-pharmacological preventative methods may include compression stockings or raising the foot of the bed by 10 cm.

Drugs

The palliation of symptoms of respiratory distress is extremely important for well-being. In an increasing proportion of cases NIV is being used for palliation, but in selected situations and for patients who cannot tolerate NIV drug therapy can be very effective, but carries the inevitable concern that it may further depress respiratory drive. However, this must not prevent the adequate palliation of symptoms, as long as patient choice is considered.

- Lorazepam:
  - 0.5–2 mg sub-lingually.
  - Very helpful for acute exacerbations of dyspnoea for whatever reason.
  - MND patients with raised pCO_2 can be very sensitive to relatively small doses of benzodiazepines.
- Morphine:
  - 5 mg nebulized for acute exacerbations.
  - 2.5 mg IV, subcutaneously, or transdermally every 4 hours for more continuous symptoms.
- Chlorpromazine:
  - 12.5 mg every 4–12 hours (can be given rectally).
  - For terminal restlessness only.

- Oxygen:
  - Rarely indicated. MND patients with raised CO_2 can also be extremely sensitive to exogenous oxygen which can dramatically reduce respiratory drive, thereby exacerbating hypercapnia.
  - However, some patients find oxygen helpful to relieve dyspnoea.

Orthopnoea

- In the absence of cardiac failure, breathlessness when lying flat is a cardinal sign of diaphragmatic weakness.
- Breathlessness with immersion in water, such as in a swimming pool, may be the first manifestation.
- A change in sleeping position, initially to sleeping on one side, but graduating to using pillows as a prop, should be viewed as a sign of incipient diaphragmatic weakness.
- Numerous studies have demonstrated that orthopnoea is the best predictor of both sleep-disordered breathing and a good response to NIV.
- Measurement of FVC both sitting and lying is an essential part of routine clinical assessment in a specialist MND clinic.
- Rarely, patients may complain of breathlessness which is present on sitting up and relieved by recumbency (known as playtpnoea). This may be due to axial and abdominal weakness leading to the patient 'folding up' when sitting, effectively reducing diaphragmatic mobility and vital capacity.

Prevention of respiratory infections

Although there has been very little systematic research, it is our clinical observation that the rate of aspiration pneumonia, even in patients who clearly do not have a competent airway, is lower than might be anticipated. However, a chest infection is a potentially devastating complication for patients with MND and preventive measures can be taken:

- Identification of at risk groups:
  - LMN-predominant pattern of weakness with loss of ability to cough and clear secretions.
  - Rapid weight loss and general debility.
  - Co-morbidities such as chronic lung disease.
- Maintenance of good nutrition with early PEG before weight loss occurs (see Chapter 10).
- Early institution of NIV.
- Avoidance of aspiration by change in diet to thickened drinks and non-particulate foods (see Chapter 10).
- Elevation of bed head at night.
- Management of inadequate cough reflex:
  - Manual abdominal thrusts from carer (taught by physiotherapist).
  - 'Breath-stacking': manual insufflation using a bag and mask prior to the cough. An NIV machine can also be used in this way to passively expand the lungs.
  - A mechanical insufflator-exsufflator ('cough-assist' device) can also be used. These are expensive and their exact role in MND patients is still being established.
- Early use of antibiotics for upper respiratory tract infections is reasonable (despite the fact that these are predominantly viral rather than bacterial), though there are no formal studies to demonstrate a lower rate of progression to lower respiratory tract infections.
- Annual influenza vaccine.

Sleep-disordered breathing

- Sleep fragmentation due to nocturnal arousals can be a early sign of impending respiratory insufficiency.
- It is important to explore the reason why the patient wakes up. There are a number of other causes for poor sleep in MND:
  - Discomfort from poor mobility.
  - Mood depression or anxiety.
  - Oral secretions.
  - Dry mouth (mouth breathing).
  - Patients will often blame a 'full bladder' for waking them up. In the context of MND this should never be accepted at face value. It is likely that the patient is waking for another reason if the symptom is of recent onset.
- A history from a bed partner is vital. They will often be aware of sleep fragmentation before the patient.
- Hypoventilation is most prominent in REM sleep (see Figure 9.1) when the diaphragm would normally do the work of breathing and other muscles are paralysed.
- Significant hypercapnia is suggested by:
  - Lack of refreshing sleep.
  - Early morning headache or mental 'grogginess'.
  - Loss of appetite in the morning.
  - Nocturia.
  - Inappropriate daytime somnolence.

Non-invasive ventilation

This consists of positive-pressure ventilation delivered via a sealed mask. The emphasis is currently on treatment of symptoms, not as a primary means of improving survival. However, a small number of clinical trials and a larger number of observational studies suggest that there is a likely to be a significant survival effect, with considerable variation between patients.

Patient selection

- NIV is generally well tolerated, but may not be suitable for every patient.
- It is likely at present to be difficult to establish NIV successfully in patients who have few or no symptoms, unless evidence emerges of significant survival benefit for early treatment.
- Rigid selection criteria have not been established and clinical practice is constantly undergoing revision in the light of experience.
- If the history suggests any symptoms of nocturnal sleep fragmentation that cannot be explained by other factors, then on empirical grounds a trial of NIV may be reasonable.
- However, we would advise that overnight oximetry is performed first to provide objective evidence of the relative contribution of respiratory muscle weakness compared to other factors.
- Alternatively, or in addition, a morning blood gas demonstrating a pCO_2 >6.5 kPa should prompt a trial of NIV in symptomatic patients.
- It is clear that patients with significant bulbar symptoms, especially flaccid paralysis, may not as a group adapt well to NIV. Inability to protect the airway is considered to be a relative contraindication to NIV. However, there are individuals even within the bulbar/corticobulbar group who can manage NIV well and who derive good symptom control.
- NIV may not be suitable for patients with frank dementia, but individual cases should be treated on their merits.

Management

- Ideally, NIV should be managed in partnership with a respiratory team with expertise in the provision of non-invasive ventilation for neuromuscular disease.
- Patients should be well informed and have realistic expectations:
  - Maintenance of well-being and symptom control are the main goals.
  - The most beneficial effect can be expected at night, with re-establishment of restorative sleep and attendant improvement of energy and vitality during the day.
  - We discourage use of NIV during the day, though some patients inevitably find this helpful.
- Choice of system:
  - Continuous positive airway pressure ventilation (CPAP) is not generally used in MND.
  - Intermittent positive-pressure ventilation.
  - Bi-level positive-pressure ventilation, in which different levels of pressure are delivered in inspiration and expiration. This is now the most frequently used method in MND patients.

- The face or nasal mask must be a tight fit, but with care to avoid pressure sores.
- Good secretion management is important.
- Because patients with MND usually have normal lung function long-term management is often quite straightforward with little need for readjustment of ventilator settings.

Tracheostomy ventilation

Background and incidence

- It is clear that emergency tracheostomy ventilation (TV) is irreversible in the majority of cases of MND and such crises should therefore be minimized by early discussion and documentation of end-of-life choices.
- There are a number of things which influence the likelihood of patients having elective TV:
  - Patient perceptions of poor quality of life and loss of autonomy with advanced MND.
  - Physician attitudes to TV: it is very difficult for physicians to present the option of TV in a neutral way. Although this may appear to undermine patient autonomy, it has to be acknowledged that patients and their carers look to the specialist care team for guidance and information based on professional experience balanced with compassion. Patient-centred care inevitably involves professional judgments about individual personality, coping strategies, and psychological resources which will colour the way in which difficult matters such as TV are discussed.
  - Availability of local resources for specialist community based care.
  - The high financial burden (approx. £150,000 per year for community care) restricts TV to those with independent financial resources in societies without universal health care coverage. Even where such coverage exists, as in the UK NHS, home care with TV is likely to be viewed as non-standard and will require a special application for funding.
  - Disease progression: tracheostomy is more likely to occur with acute respiratory presentations before the diagnosis of MND has been made, rather than in more typical forms of ALS in which there is a more predictable rate of decline.
- The rate of tracheostomy in MND is generally about 2–3%, although higher in some countries (Japan, 30%; Italy, 10%).
- There is no evidence to suggest at present that the rate of tracheostomy ventilation is increasing as a result of greater use of NIV. In fact, it is possible that a more controlled and less crisis-driven approach to the management of symptomatic and terminal respiratory failure in MND could make TV less likely.

Effect on natural history

- Our understanding of the natural history of MND in patients with TV is incomplete.
- It is clear that if ventilation is artificially supported the 'multisystem' nature of MND becomes manifest:
  - Many patients develop extraocular paralysis and selected data from autopsy studies typically shows generalized cerebral atrophy.
  - Assessing cognitive decline in patients who are effectively 'locked-in' is challenging. Although it is likely that the incidence of dementia is higher in these patients, even with prolonged survival with tracheostomy there appear to be at least some examples of patients with normal cognitive function despite prolonged invasive ventilation.

- The underlying neurodegenerative process continues until it ultimately involves neurological control of circulatory homeostasis. Circulatory collapse is a common cause of death with TV.
- Survival varies enormously, reflecting that patients selected for TV will be a heterogeneous group. An important determinant is whether patient selection is slanted towards those with slow progression. The application of TV as crisis management for terminal respiratory failure is likely to result in a poor outcome (50% survival at one year in one study). Other series with slower progressing patients report an average survival of 4 years.
- Complications of tracheostomy:
  - fistula
  - infection
  - tracheal stenosis
  - pneumothorax
  - subcutaneous emphysema.
- The determinants of a 'positive outcome' when home-based TV is chosen are considered to be:
  - A highly motivated patient with slowly progressive MND.
  - An ability to communicate and perform some activities of daily living.
  - A clear appreciation of the available options.
  - Appropriate care from family and/or care teams.
- The minimum requirements to set up home-based tracheostomy include:
  - The availability of in-hospital training for families and other carers.
  - A designated case manager to develop funding for a care package and to coordinate the establishment of a multidisciplinary team.
  - Preparation of an appropriate physical environment at home, which may include building work. Building regulations may require the construction of an appropriate emergency exit. Electrical provision for ventilator, suction equipment, adjustable bed, etc.
  - A policy for coping with loss of electrical supply, e.g. battery-operated backup ventilator in the event of a power cut.
  - 24-hour support from equipment manufacturers.
  - Availability of respite for carers.
  - An advance statement of: (a) the patient's wishes in the event of sudden cardiorespiratory decline; (b) under what circumstances they would wish TV to be terminated.
- Carer burden is very high. More than half of carers report that TV is a major burden and a similar number that their own health has suffered as a result of their caring role.

Terminal weaning is legal in the UK. However, it is likely that the medical team will need the support of an independent medical and legal opinion, or an ethics committee, in some circumstances. Terminal weaning should be done under the cover of intravenous opioid analgesia.

Suggested approach to discussing request for tracheostomy

- It is the practice in some centres to routinely discuss TV as one of a range of options. Other centres discuss it on an individual patient-by-patient basis.
- TV should be acknowledged as a legitimate option in MND, but with an emphasis on patient selection and a frank discussion of the factors outlined here which are associated with a 'positive outcome'.
- Establish the patient's motivation for seeking tracheostomy, specifically exploring whether it is driven by:
  - unrealistic expectations of advances in treatment for MND (e.g. by stem cell therapy)
  - the wish to stay alive for the benefit of others, e.g. young children
  - fear of an unpleasant sudden death, e.g. by 'choking'.
- Explore the patient's understanding of the implications of TV for disease progression:
  - Motor weakness will continue to progress and for the majority of patients who elect to have TV will graduate to a 'locked-in' state.
  - There is a significant chance of major cognitive involvement with time.
  - Communication will become increasingly challenging and even eye movements may fail.
  - Survival will still be limited, with a significant chance of overwhelming pulmonary infection (e.g. in an Italian series the survival post-TV averaged one year).
- As discussed, physician attitudes to the appropriateness of TV in the management of MND vary considerably. However, complete refusal by the care team to discuss or consider tracheostomy as an option is inappropriate and will provoke a very negative reaction in some patients, who may then resort to legal measures in an attempt to try and 'force' medical intervention. We strongly advocate a balanced and honest discussion of the implications of TV.

Further reading

Bourke SC, Tomlinson M, Williams TL, Bullock RE, Shaw PJ, Gibson GJ (2006). Effects of non-invasive ventilation on survival and quality of life in patients with amyotrophic lateral sclerosis: a randomised controlled trial. *Lancet Neurol* 5,140–147.

Nutrition

Introduction

Nutrition is important in MND for quality of life and maintaining general health and energy levels. Malnutrition is common in MND and it is an independent prognostic factor for survival.

Assessment, monitoring, and management of nutritional status should continue throughout the course of the disease. A multidisciplinary team based approach is essential.

Causes of weight loss in MND

Weight loss is multifactorial in most cases. Contributing factors include:
- Reduced intake:
  - Dysphagia and fear of choking.
  - Physical disability, e.g. upper limb weakness leading to dependence on others for food preparation and feeding and a reduction in snacking.
- Increased calorific requirements and hypermetabolism.
- Muscle atrophy.
- Psychological factors, e.g. reduced appetite with depression and cognitive impairment.
- Social embarrassment.
- Recurrent chest infections.

Assessment of nutritional status

Assessment and monitoring of nutritional status should continue throughout the course of the disease and involves all members of the multidisciplinary team.

- History:
  - symptoms or consequences of dysphagia (see p. 138)
  - dietary history including details of calorie intake, textures of food and liquids, portion size, and meal duration
  - measured weight loss or clothes feeling loose.
- Examination
  - weakness of facial muscles, tongue, and palate movement
  - facial and jaw reflexes
  - dentition
  - weakness of upper limbs
  - posture, e.g. position of head and neck
  - saliva
  - dysarthria.
- Specific measures
  - weight and percentage weight loss
  - Body Mass Index (weight in kg/height in m^2)
  - calculation of caloric requirements.

Problems in any of these areas should prompt a review of current nutritional management. Weight loss of 10% or more and BMI ≤ 18.5 kg/m^2 are significant indicators of malnutrition.

Dysphagia

Approximately one third of patients with MND initially present with bulbar symptoms and most typical ALS patients will eventually develop difficulties in this area. The pattern of abnormality will reflect the relative degree of upper motor neuron and lower motor neuron involvement. Dysarthria (see Chapter 8) almost always precedes swallowing problems which usually arise gradually and become more troublesome as muscle weakness and incoordination progress. The process of choking on food is extremely distressing to patients and carers but they can be reassured that it is virtually never a direct cause of death.

Symptoms of dysphagia
- The earliest symptoms include occasional choking or coughing with liquids, specific difficulty swallowing medication, or simply a heightened awareness of the swallowing process.
- Leakage of food or liquids from the mouth and associated drooling.
- Reduced swallowing frequency due to increased effort and muscle fatigue.
- Difficulty chewing food and moving it around the mouth.
- Nasal regurgitation causing a 'gurgly' or 'wet' voice.
- Coughing or choking on food or liquids.
- Sensation that 'something is stuck' when swallowing.

Stages of swallowing
- Oral preparation:
  chewing and compressing food to form a bolus depends on coordination of the lips, tongue, mastication muscles and adequate saliva.
- Oral phase:
  voluntary transfer of bolus, using the tongue, towards the pharynx to initiate reflex swallow.
- Pharyngeal phase:
  reflex stage involving a number of coordinated muscular actions to prevent bolus from entering the nasal cavity or larynx and to propel bolus towards and into the oesophagus.
- Oesophageal phase:
  reflex stage where bolus passes from the upper oesophageal sphincter to the stomach.

Any of these stages can be affected in MND if there is weakness or spasticity of the relevant muscles. Spasticity of the cricopharyngeal sphincter can also prevent the passage of the bolus into the oesophagus.

Consequences of dysphagia
- Weight loss.
- Fatigue.
- Constipation.
- Loss of appetite.
- Anxiety when eating with others.
- Loss of well-being.
- Recurrent chest infections.

Assessment of patients with dysphagia

Initial bedside evaluation

- Neurological examination to assess the degree of upper and lower motor neuron involvement:
  - Jaw and other facial jerks.
  - Movement of the palate.
  - Stiffness and reduced mobility of the tongue.
  - Assessment of tongue wasting and weakness.
  - Presence of saliva and food residue in the pharyngeal folds.
  - The gag reflex is rarely helpful in this context, and should be avoided.
- Observe the patient swallowing a small amount of liquid, looking for evidence of:
  - choking
  - coughing
  - change in voice quality
  - spillage from the mouth
  - excessive number of swallows required to clear the mouth.

Speech and language therapist assessment

- If swallowing problems are suspected the patient should be assessed by a speech and language therapist.
- Specialist assessment will include taking a full history to identify relevant symptoms and problem liquids or foods, examination, and assessment of swallow with a variety of liquids and food textures.

Investigations

It is rarely necessary to perform detailed investigation such as video-fluoroscopy or modified barium swallow to guide feeding regimes and determine risk of aspiration.

General dietary management

Nutritional management is often coordinated by the dietitian and speech and language therapist working together.

Oral intake

Intake sufficient to meet the patient's metabolic needs will vary according to changing requirements throughout the disease.

- Increase calorie intake with energy-dense meals and snack/food fortification.
- Modification of food and liquid texture according to swallowing problems, e.g. thickened liquids, soft food, pureed food.
- Prescription of supplement drinks or puddings.

Specific advice or adaptations

Optimize swallowing ability and safe oral intake.

- Management of oral secretions.
- Take small bites or sips.
- Avoid trigger foods, e.g. lettuce and other raw vegetables; dry, crumbly biscuits and cakes; mixed textures such as a thin soup with chunks of meat; hard food such as nuts or dry toast; spicy food; stringy food such as bacon rind.
- Swallow techniques, e.g. head turn, chin tuck, repeated swallow to clear the mouth.
- Specialist equipment to aid feeding, e.g. adaptive cutlery, mobile arm supports.
- Posture, e.g. sitting upright with adequate head and trunk support.
- Sucking ice prior to eating to reduce bulbar muscle spasticity.
- Decrease unnecessary energy expenditure through adaptations or assistance.
- Education of patient and carer.

Artificial nutrition

When oral intake and other adaptations fail to maintain adequate nutritional status, or swallowing deteriorates to a stage where there is significant risk of aspiration, alternative routes of nutritional intake should be activated. At this stage enteral nutrition strategies should already be fully explored and put in place. It is entirely legitimate to place an enteral feeding tube in a patient without significant dysphagia, but who is either very likely to develop swallowing problems or who will benefit from enteral nutrition because of other factors associated with malnutrition listed previously.

Enteral nutrition methods

Percutaneous endoscopic gastrostomy (PEG) or percutaneous endoscopic jejunostomy (PEJ)

PEG is the most common method of providing non-oral enteral nutrition. The procedure involves insertion of a tube through the abdominal wall into the stomach (gastrostomy) or small intestine (jejunostomy) under endoscopic guidance and requires a small amount of sedation. A working partnership between the MND team and a gastroenterologist with an interest in this area is important as MND patients differ significantly in their risk profile from other patients undergoing this procedure (e.g. stroke).

Radiologically inserted gastrostomy (RIG)

This approach may be used if the endoscopic approach fails, in patients in the terminal phase, or in those with poor respiratory function (FVC <50%). In some centres this is the technique of choice. As with PEG, identification of an interventional radiologist with an interest and particular experience in this technique to develop a long term partnership with the MND team is the ideal pathway. Techniques for the procedure vary, but generally sedation is not required and patients can remain upright. Oral contrast medium is given before the procedure. The gastrostomy is inserted under radiologic guidance.

Nasogastric tube (NGT)

Long-term use of this method is not advised, but it may be useful for short periods. It is generally more uncomfortable for patients, and can increase oral secretions or lead to aspiration. Easy displacement and repeated replacement can be distressing and may cause nasal trauma. In our practice this is reserved as a last resort for patients in the terminal phase of their illness who refuse a PEG or who have presented too late to benefit.

Parenteral nutrition

This is very uncommon in MND. It may be used in extreme situations if it is not possible to provide enteral nutrition through the routes already described. It involves intravenous delivery of nutritional solution.

Benefits of PEG or RIG

- Prevention of malnutrition through adequate nutritional intake.
- Prevention of dehydration.
- Alternative route for medication.
- Reduced anxiety and pressure to achieve sufficient oral intake.

- Improved quality of life.
- Patients can continue to eat and drink for enjoyment.

Complications of PEG or RIG

Adverse events are unusual but commoner ones include:
- Bleeding from wound (transient, and rarely significant).
- Post-procedure ileus (usually <24 hours).
- Wound tenderness (sometimes requires repositioning of fastener).
- Wound infections – early and late (usually respond to a short course of oral antibiotics after swab).
- Procedure-related mortality.
- Gastrointestinal symptoms, e.g. diarrhoea, abdominal pain, gastric reflux.
- Tubes can become blocked or displaced.
- Refeeding syndrome: this should be very rare in the context of MND. Severely malnourished patients can develop a constellation of metabolic derangements as normal nutritional status is re-established. Hypophosphataemia is the commonest abnormality. In at-risk patients careful monitoring of biochemical tests is advisable.

Timing of PEG or RIG insertion

This depends on a number of factors, however the earlier the gastrostomy is placed, the more successful the procedure. In historical case series, in which the practice was to insert a PEG in the more advanced stage of MND, there was a conspicuously high early mortality (25% in the first month). This was largely attributable to the natural history of the disease and a clear argument for early intervention.

Ideal approach:
- Discussion about gastrostomy placement should be introduced at the earliest opportunity with patients likely to require this intervention during their disease. A particular group that benefits greatly from early PEG is the progressive bulbar palsy subgroup, often elderly women with maintained limb strength despite rapidly progressive dysarthria.
- Patients are naturally reluctant to undergo the procedure and it is important that they understand the risks associated with delay or refusal.
- As long as patients have been adequately informed, not having a PEG tube inserted is a legitimate choice. In a minority of patients this undoubtedly complicates the terminal phase of MND and makes an NGT much more likely. Other patients appear to manage significant dysphagia remarkably well and continue to eat and drink without major complications.
- Given the risks associated with performing the procedure if the vital capacity is below 50% of predicted, it is unjustifiable to delay if there is a clear indication of decline from successive measures of respiratory function.
- Patients should be prepared for PEG by a joint consultation with the MDT in which they are introduced to the procedure, shown a PEG tube, and informed about the risks and benefits of the procedure.

- This is an ideal time to introduce discussion of an advance directive, including the patient's wishes in the unlikely event of sudden cardiorespiratory arrest.
- It is not sufficient to rely on measuring FVC sitting upright as this will miss incipient diaphragmatic weakness. Lying and sitting FVC should be recorded. If both are above 60% the risk of complications from the procedure is low. If either measure is below 60% it is advisable to perform blood gas estimation and, in selected cases, overnight oximetry. If there are clear indications of respiratory failure (see Chapter 9), advice should be sought from respiratory medicine colleagues so that NIV can be instituted prior to the PEG/RIG procedure.

Management of enteral nutrition

Gastrostomy insertion should be coordinated closely with the community dietitian who will be responsible for ongoing nutritional management. They will continue to determine the patient's nutritional requirements and the most appropriate method and rate of feeding.

Options for feeding include:
- bolus feeds during the day via syringe (performed by patient or carer)
- continuous feed via portable electric pump (can run overnight).

It is important to gradually increase the volume of fluid or feed through the gastrostomy to avoid gastrointestinal complications. It is also important for the patient's primary carer to be involved in discussions about enteral feeding as they will be essential in the ongoing management and will require education and specific training.

Further reading

Heffernan C, Jenkinson C, Holmes T, *et al.* (2004). Nutritional management in MND/ALS patients: an evidence based review. *Amyotrophic Lateral Sclerosis*, 5, 72–83.

Disability management

Introduction

Disability is an umbrella term that is generally used to describe limitation of function experienced as a result of a disease or illness. In 1980 the WHO developed the ICIDH (International Classification of Impairments, Disabilities, and Handicaps) to define and classify the impact of disease on the individual (see Figure 11.1).

Classification

- Impairment – impact of disease process on the body.
- Disability – impact of impairments on functional performance and activities.
- Handicap – impact of impairments and disabilities on a person in society.

This classification system was revised and published as the WHO IC (International Classification of Function) in 2001. This revised model use a biopsychosocial approach and acknowledges the additional impact o factors other than the disease process on a person's functional abilities These are described as contextual factors and include personal, physica environmental, and social factors (see Figure 11.2).

This framework not only provides a structure for identifying areas o limitation, but also the areas in which changes can be made to increase functional ability. This is particularly important in motor neuron disease where functional ability is continuously changing and where treatment are limited. For example, despite progressive impairments physical aid may be used to enable independence in daily tasks which would otherwise be impossible without another person's assistance.

In MND there are often specific windows of opportunity for intervention Aids can be introduced or environments changed at a time when a person develops further impairment and is no longer able to perform particula tasks. However, these adaptations may only be useable at that level o impairment, and when there is further progression they may no longe enable the same level of independence. These windows are often short sometimes only a few months, and therefore there is the need for a rapid response to facilitate ongoing independence.

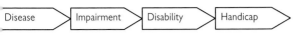

Fig. 11.1 WHO schema for classification of disability stages.

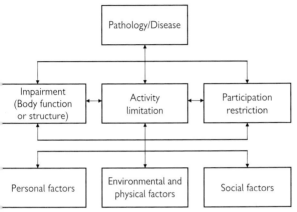

Fig. 11.2 Factors which combine in the interaction between individuals and their disease.

Life goal planning

- A process that identifies a person's lifestyle priorities.
- Focuses management on those areas to achieve identified goals.
- In most rehabilitation settings there is a formal goal setting process, which facilitates the patient, their relatives, and the multidisciplinary team in planning future management.
- The patient is asked to identify the areas of their life that are most important and, in conjunction with the team, they agree on particular goals to be achieved in a designated time period.
- Goals may be set at the impairment level, but are most commonly set at the activity or participation levels.
- Goal planning often occurs in a more informal manner in many MND services with the team taking a rather more directive role, highlighting specific issues that will be encountered in the future.
- Enables decision-making in areas such as where the person wants to live, whether they want to undergo particular interventions, and also end-of-life matters.
- Key lifestyle areas include:
  - employment
  - relationships
  - accommodation
  - finances
  - personal care
  - mobility
  - driving
  - leisure activities
  - religion or spirituality.
- Issues particular to MND include:
  - feeding and nutrition
  - breathing
  - end-of-life matters such as antibiotic use, hospital admission, and place of death.

Role of exercise

- Whether to exercise is a question frequently asked by patients. Despite suggestions that 'athleticism' may be a risk factor for MND, there is no evidence that taking exercise either increases or decreases the rate of disease progression.
- An exercise program is a way for people with MND to take an active and positive role in maintaining well-being and is important for preventing secondary disability.
- Programmed exercise or physiotherapy will not improve muscle strength. However, exercise in moderation can promote:
  - Flexibility: important in maintaining muscle length, a full range of movement around joints, and in preventing contractures.
  - Good balance: falls can be minimized by good walking techniques, which can be taught by a physiotherapist.
  - General health and well-being: exercise can help improve quality of life, minimize fatigue, and promote good sleep hygiene.
  - A sense of physical independence at a time when functions are recognized to be failing. In contrast, patients with rapidly progressive disease may find exercise demoralizing so advice has to be appropriate to the individual.
  - Mood: can help with depression and fatigue and improve sense of energy.
  - Reduced pain and spasticity.
  - Weight management: this may be helpful in the early phase of MND when a reduction in activity can promote weight gain. However, actively trying to lose weight is never recommended for people living with MND.
- Any exercise programme will need to be monitored and adaptations made to
  - frequency
  - intensity
  - duration.

Role of the physiotherapist

A physiotherapist may provide input at all stages of the disease, including:

- in the early stages of disease:
  - assessment of motor power, joint range of movement, and functional abilities to give the patient confidence to exercise
  - provision of mobility aids
  - instruction in how to exercise safely and effectively
  - support in teaching passive exercises to carers.
- in the interim stages:
  - re assessment of motor function and exercise programme
  - pain relief measures such as ice, heat, and acupuncture
  - assessment of chest function; teaching breath stacking (see Chapter 9)
  - assessment of aids and replacement if necessary
  - advice on moving and handling for all transfers
  - advice about splinting and positioning.

- during the terminal phase:
  - general re-assessment of physical and functional abilities
  - introduction of assisted and passive stretches
  - care of oedematous feet and hands; use of pressure bandages
  - reassessment of aids and advice on withdrawal of aids where necessary
  - advice to carer and other professionals on positioning, moving, and handling
  - advice about chest management, implications of deterioration, and use of assisted cough technique (see Chapter 9).

Types of exercise

Appropriate exercises for MND patients include:

- in the early stages:
  - walking
  - swimming, providing respiratory function is adequate
  - cycling, providing there are no problems with stopping and balance
  - gym, with advice and guidance
- during interim stage:
  - walking, with aids if necessary
  - static exercise bike
  - home exercise programme, particularly stretching exercises
  - deep breathing exercises/breath stacking
- during the terminal phase:
  - assisted and passive stretches
  - care of shoulder and other joints
  - assisted cough chest expansion exercises.

Driving

All drivers have a personal responsibility to ensure they are safe to drive and are fully in control of their vehicle. Thus the same factors apply to someone with neurological disease that renders them unable to drive safely as those that prohibit driving whilst under the influence of drugs or alcohol. It is not primarily a medical decision that prevents someone with MND from driving and MND is not on the list of conditions that automatically prohibit driving. However, patients with newly diagnosed MND do have to inform the Driver and Vehicle Licensing Agency (DVLA) and failure to do so could potentially lead to a fine (see Appendix 1).

For most people driving a car is a key element of their independence and they will wish to maintain this function for as long as possible. The vast majority of people in our experience are extremely careful and insightful and stop driving well before the period when there is significant risk of an accident.

Major warning signs

- Evidence of clinically obvious cognitive impairment. Being able to multi-task is an essential skill for driving. Given the lack of insight associated with frontotemporal dementia, it can be difficult to persuade someone that they are a risk and it is critical to involve family members in ensuring that access to the vehicle is restricted. This may necessitate formal cognitive testing and the involvement of colleagues expert in determining capacity, e.g. an old-age psychiatrist.
- Concerns expressed by family members should always be taken very seriously. In addition to often being the first indication of cognitive impairment, such concerns may rarely reflect denial on the part of the patient. It may be more acceptable for some patients to be advised by the doctor that driving should stop.
- Rapidly progressive disease. It may be difficult for the patient to appreciate the impact of rapidly changing disability on the ability to drive.
- Significant sleep fragmentation in otherwise amubulant patients with the attendant risk of daytime somnolence.

Adaptations to the vehicle

If the barrier to driving is purely physical, caused by weakness of specific muscle groups, there are many adaptations which can be made to the car to enable the continuation of driving in a safe and comfortable manner.

- Hand or arm weakness:
  - Car keys can be adapted by enlarging the grip to enable more leverage on the key head.
  - A steering knob can be fitted to the rim of the steering wheel.
  - Automatic 'press button' ignition.
  - Indicators, horn, lights changed to foot control or placed within finger reach of the steering wheel.
  - Moving the hand brake to the driver's strongest side.
  - Joy-stick steering.
  - Automatic transmission.
  - A steering panel can be controlled by the foot.
  - Changing the seat belt to a harness.

- Lower-limb weakness:
  - Automatic transmission which does not require a clutch.
  - Hand controls for brake and accelerator.
- Access and transfers to vehicle:
  - Swivel or sliding seat aid.
  - Wide doors.
  - Leg-lifter to help lift the legs into the car.
  - Sliding board.
  - Use of handling belt.
  - Hoists.
  - There are also specially adapted cars which accommodate a wheelchair.

Sources of information

Before thinking about purchasing a new car or making adaptations to an old one, advice can be sought from a local Mobility Advice & Vehicle Information Service (MAVIS). The Department of Transport has lists of centres which are located across the country. If adaptations are made to a vehicle extra lessons or training is recommended, particularly if the adaptations involve foot controls.

Insurance

- It is mandatory to inform insurers of a significant new medical diagnosis.
- Motor insurance is vital. There are many companies which specialise in insuring people with a disability.
- However, it is important for patients to shop carefully and be fully informed of all exclusions clauses before taking out adequate motor insurance.

Blue Badges

- People living with MND may apply for a Blue Badge. This scheme provides a range of parking concessions for people who have severe mobility problems and cannot assess public transport with ease.
- The badge belongs to the person and not the car, and so can be transferred to any vehicle in which the person with a disability is travelling.
- It applies to on-street parking, free use of pay and display bays, and parking meters.
- It exempts badge holders from time restrictions.
- It allows parking of up to three hours on a single or double yellow line, providing no obstruction is caused or other restrictions are in place.
- It exempts people from the Congestion Charge in London. The badge holder does have to register with Transport for London (TfL) at least 10 days prior to their journey. They must also pay a one-off registration fee.
- The Blue Badge Scheme does not apply to off-street parking, private roads, or airports.
- This scheme runs throughout the United Kingdom although there may be slight differences for people living in Wales, Scotland, and Northern Ireland.
- The Blue Badge may also be used throughout Europe.

Motability Scheme
- Allows people with a disability to use their mobility allowance to acquire a new car, wheelchair, or scooter:
  - Contract Hire covers all service and maintenance, insurance, and breakdown cover for a period of three years.
  - Hire Purchase allows the individual to buy their car outright.
- To be eligible people must be receiving the Higher Rate Mobility Component (HRMC) of the Disability Living Allowance (DLA) or War Pensioner's Mobility Supplement (WPMS).
- People who are claiming allowances under the DS1500 are not eligible for this scheme.

Air travel

Many patients with MND ask advice about long-haul travel. Given the progressive nature of the disease, there are clearly important issues about the timing of such journeys to minimize risk.

Insurance

- Having comprehensive travel insurance is the single most important issue. A brief medical consultation can run to several hundred pounds, and a short stay in hospital can run to many thousands. This is a particularly severe issue in North America.
- Many travel insurance companies will cover MND patients but, crucially, not for MND-related medical care. For those with significant disability it is hard to prove that hospital admission or other medical care was in no way related to, or more importantly, not complicated or prolonged by the diagnosis of MND, and insurance companies may then refuse to pay. There may be a significant financial premium attached to ensuring that MND is fully covered.
- When travelling within the EU, a valid EHIC card (formerly known as the E111) is essential.

The practicalities of foreign travel

- The UK could perform a lot better in terms of disabled access, but there are many countries with less well developed facilities.
- Liaison with airlines and airport authorities will ensure that anyone with a disability is given preferential treatment. People with disabilities now have EU-specified 'rights to fly'.
- Security regulations about the volume of liquid allowed in hand luggage are a problem for people traveling with enteral feed. A covering letter from the clinic team will help but it is worth contacting airport security before traveling (including stop-over airports). The number for disability facilities information at Heathrow is 020 8745 6155.
- Specialized equipment (e.g. NIV) may have to be cleared through security separately.
- It is also important to advise people to think about the on-board arrangements, particularly for eating, drinking, and using the lavatory during the journey.
- At the other end, will there be help with luggage? What if bags are lost or delayed - would there be vital equipment or medication in it?
- Patients with communication difficulties should travel with a Lightwriter™ if they use one. Point It!™ picture books for travellers are full of pictures of food, household items, buildings, vehicles, clothing, etc. and can ensure efficient and rapid communication (www.graf-editions.de/pointit). These can be obtained from Cordee Distributors (sales@cordee.co.uk).

Prevention of deep vein thrombosis

- MND patients with increased physical disability and restricted leg movements have a higher risk of DVT during long-haul travel.
- Prevention:
  - Wearing full-length compression stockings.
  - Aspirin 75 mg for three days either side of air travel is reasonable, though there is no clear evidence base for this.
  - Maintain good hydration.

Travelling with NIV

- The level of oxygen inside pressurized commercial aircraft cabins is equivalent to that at about 2500 m. In theory this could cause problems in a patient with significant diaphragm weakness, significant breathlessness at rest, or orthopnoea.
- For those MND patients already established on NIV, the main issue is ensuring uninterrupted power supply if needed. Taking a spare battery and appropriate adaptors is recommended. Advance discussion with the airline and leaving more time to clear security are advisable.

Mobility issues

- Virtually all patients with MND will develop difficulty with mobility at some point.
- For some this may be the first sign of MND, whereas for others with more slowly progressive disease mainly affecting their upper limbs this may only occur late in the disease process.
- Mobility in the broadest sense includes all transfers, walking indoors and outdoors, and accessing the community.
- It may be affected by a variety of factors (see Table 11.1).
- Due to the potentially complex causes of mobility problems, multidisciplinary assessment is essential to identify the most appropriate management plan.
- Considering again the WHO ICF, interventions may be at the impairment, activity, or participation levels; with the introduction of a range of physical, environmental, and social factors (see Table 11.2).
- Goals of intervention include:
  - maintaining independent mobility
  - mobility with assistance
  - preventing falls and injury
  - preventing social isolation.

Falls

Disease progression is associated with increased risk and frequency of falls, which can have significant consequences.

- Causes:
  - Leg weakness, unable to negotiate obstacles.
  - Arm weakness, preventing automatic saving mechanisms.
  - Spasticity, limiting fast corrective movements to stop falling.
- Complications:
  - Leg fractures can result in long-term reduction in mobility due to secondary muscle wasting from disuse.
  - Arm or hand fractures can result in inability to carry out daily activities.
  - Head injury.
  - Inability to get up from the floor, pressure sores, rhabdomyolysis.

Table 11.1 Causes of reduced mobility

Physical	Lower-limb and trunk weakness
	Upper-limb weakness limiting use of mobility aids
	Spasticity
Cognitive or psychological	Cognitive impairments
	Anxiety or depression
	Reduced confidence
Environmental	Home setup, including stairs and space to accommodate mobility aids
	Outdoor terrain
Social	Access to private or public transport
	Access to buildings for work or leisure activities

Table 11.2 Examples of interventions

Orthotics	Ankle foot orthoses
	Custom-made shoes
Walking aids	Walking sticks or poles
	Crutches
	Walking frames, wheeled or static
Spasticity management	Medication
	Stretching programme
Aids for transfers	Slide board
	Disc turners
	Hoists
Alternative mobility aids	Manual wheelchair
	Powered wheelchair
Psychological	Support for altered mood
	Prompts or set up for cognitive impairment
Home adaptations	Installation of rails for support
	Removal of potential obstacles
	Stair-lift, ramp access
	Widening doorways
	One-level living
Social environment adaptations	As for home adaptations, but in shared community settings
	Vehicle adaptations

Mobility aids

Orthotics

An orthosis is a device that is applied to the body to facilitate function; they may also be known as splints or supports. All orthoses add extra weight to a limb and some patients find them too cumbersome to use regularly.

- The most commonly used orthosis in MND is an ankle-foot orthosis (AFO) to compensate for foot drop.
- Prefabricated AFOs are available in standard sizes for the right or left foot. They are less expensive than custom-made models and are useful in evaluating benefit or in rapidly changing situations.
- Custom-made orthoses allow intimate fit to a patient's limb, are easily adapted to provide optimal support, and are often lighter in weight than 'off the shelf' models.
- More discrete supports include the 'foot-up' splint and the more expensive Silicone AFO. These are useful with mild to moderate foot drop, but may not provide sufficient floor clearance during walking when weakness progresses.

Walking aids

A wide variety of walking aids are available and provision should follow assessment by a neurological physiotherapist. It is important that the appropriate aid is the correct size and is used in the correct manner to optimise mobility and safety.

- Walking sticks are often one of the first aids to be used. These may be standard or may have contoured hand grips, e.g. Fisher sticks.
- Some people choose to use commercially available walking poles instead of walking sticks as they are perceived as less stigmatising.
- One or two crutches may also be used if preferred or if more support is needed.
- Walking frames come in a range of designs, from standard Zimmer frames to those with wheels and an incorporated basket and seat. The type of frame chosen is often dependent on personal preference and the activities for which the frame will be used.

Spasticity management (see Chapter 8)

- In some forms of MND spasticity is a major feature and this can have a significant impact on mobility.
- Increased muscle tone can result in abnormal positioning of the foot or leg during walking, resulting in an unbalanced gait.
- Medication should be prescribed cautiously as some patients use their extensor spasticity to weight-bear and reducing it may reveal the underlying weakness.

Wheelchairs and seating systems

Wheelchairs are essential when walking becomes too difficult or impossible. Their use can enhance quality of life, improve safety, and promote independence in functional activities.

- Initially a patient might use a wheelchair on an intermittent basis for travelling longer distances before going on to rely on it for all mobility.

- A wheelchair or seating system will include specific features to provide pressure relief when sitting for long periods and postural support.
- Wheelchairs are generally provided by the local wheelchair service after comprehensive assessment to identify the most appropriate model for the patient based on:
  - physical and cognitive impairments
  - rate of disease progression
  - daily activities
  - lifestyle and personal goals
  - home environment
  - available resources.
- Referral to specialist seating or posture services may be necessary for more complex management, particularly for those with PLS.

Wheelchairs can generally be divided into manual and powered chairs, with or without a tilt mechanism:

- **Standard manual wheelchairs** are the most basic, with limited adjustability, and are generally the first to be used on an intermittent basis. They will either be designed to be pushed by an attendant or to allow self-propulsion. They are relatively portable and most can be folded for transportation or storage. These chairs do not provide sufficient support for a full-time wheelchair user.
- **Lightweight manual wheelchairs** are occasionally provided in the case of a more slowly progressive disease with predominant lower-limb involvement. These are easier to self propel and can be adjusted to provide the most supportive and efficient posture for manoeuvrability.
- **Powered wheelchairs** can enable a person to be independent even though they are unable to walk or self-propel a manual wheelchair. There are many different models that vary in size, price, and suitability for indoor or outdoor use and additional functions. They can be controlled using standard joysticks, switch arrays, and head-switches, among others.
- **Tilt-in-space frame wheelchairs** (see Figure 11.3) allow rotation in space for pressure management and increased postural support. This mechanism is available for both manual and powered wheelchairs. The seat and backrest maintain their positions in relation to each other, usually 90°, and the complete seating system tilts back on the wheelchair base. This adaptation is useful when posture deteriorates during the day, but still allows an upright position at other times

Although using a powered wheelchair can increase independent mobility there are some disadvantages including their larger size and weight, need for more space to manoeuvre, requirement of a bigger vehicle with ramp access for transportation, and increased price.

Wheelchair cushions

- Most wheelchairs do not have integral cushions and these must be supplied separately according to the amount of support and pressure relief needed.
- As a general principle, the more time a person spends in their wheelchair the more support and pressure relief they need.

- The most basic cushion is composed of foam and can be used for up to four hours a day.
- Cushions providing more pressure relief are made from gel, fluid, air, or a combination of materials. These cushions aim to distribute pressure over a large area to reduce the effect of high pressure over susceptible areas such as the sacrum or ischial tuberosities which could cause pressure sores. Some cushions reduce shear forces, which can also damage soft tissues.
- The composition of some pressure-relieving cushions may cause the user to feel unstable, particularly if they have reduced sitting balance, and often a compromise is needed.

Wheelchair adaptations

- A wheelchair will have footrests to support the feet and these should be positioned appropriately for the user's size and correct posture in sitting.
- Foot straps may be added if it difficult to maintain foot position due to weakness or spasticity.
- Additional support may be needed as weakness increases and adaptations such as a headrest or lateral trunk supports can usually be added to the user's current wheelchair.

Specialist seating

- Those with significantly complex physical problems may require more support and pressure relief than is available in a standard wheelchair with adaptations, and a custom-made seating system may be advised.
- These are typically foam contoured or made from a matrix system.
- They are expensive and unlikely to be appropriate for those with a rapidly progressive condition with changing support needs. Therefore they tend to be more suitable for those with a more slowly progressive condition and complex postural needs.

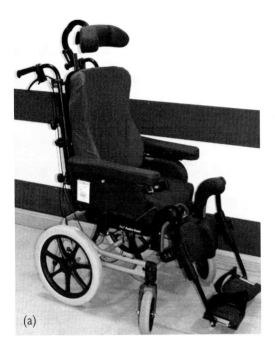

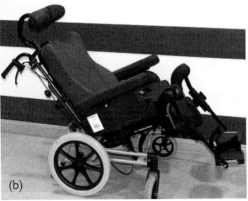

Fig. 11.3 (a) Wheelchair in standard position; (b) tilt-in-space wheelchair in 'tilt position' note the angle between wheelchair back and seat remains at 90 degrees).

Collars

- It is not uncommon for people with MND to develop head drop due to weakness of extensor muscles of the neck and back.
- Consequences:
  - Discomfort due to immobility or attempts to maintain upright posture.
  - Reduced visual field due to head position, making it difficult to see ahead and avoid obstacles, leading to risk of falls.
  - Postural instability.
  - Reduced eye contact with others.
  - Difficulty when eating and drinking.
  - Drooling of saliva.
- There are many different types of neck collar available. One particular collar may not be suitable for everyone or for all activities.
- Available collars (see Figure 11.4):
  - Soft collars, e.g. foam or filled with polystyrene balls.
  - Semi-rigid collars, e.g. Philadelphia or Aspen.
  - Headmaster collar.
  - MND Oxford collar.
  - Oxford Lees Head support.
  - Head supports and collars may be incorporated in wheelchair adaptations.
  - Custom-made collars may be required if head position is not accommodated with available collars, e.g. significant lateral flexion.
- The main aim in using a collar is to reduce the impact of head drop in daily activities.
- Disadvantages of using a collar:
  - Discomfort due to immobility.
  - Pressure points due to supports on chest or clavicles.
  - Soft collars may provide less support.
  - Circumferential collars may feel restrictive.
  - Most available collars do not provide lateral support.
  - Restriction of swallow.

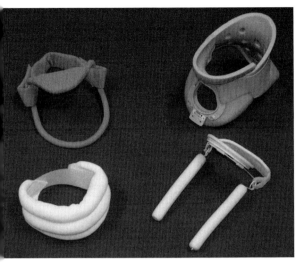

Fig. 11.4 Commonly used collars; clockwise from top left: headmaster collar, semi-rigid collar, Oxford collar, soft collar.

Mobile arm supports

- Also known as 'balanced forearm orthoses', 'balanced linkage feeders', and 'ball-bearing arm supports'. These were originally developed in the USA in the 1930s to improve function in patients with polio and severe disability from proximal upper-limb weakness.
- They give support to the arm and increase the range of movement by overcoming the mechanical disadvantage imposed by gravity.
- They can be used to aid:
  - eating
  - page turning
  - accessing a computer keyboard
  - painting, drawing, or writing.
- The provision of MAS requires a specialist assessment and can take a long time. It is important to be proactive in getting this equipment in a timely fashion.
- Patients will be reluctant to use an MAS if arm function is too good.
- Once arms and shoulders become too weak the benefit of an MAS is lost.
- Indications that mobile arm supports may be of benefit include:
  - resting the arm on the edge of the table and using it as a pivot during eating
  - bringing the head down low to meet the hands during eating
  - eating very slowly and tiring quickly.
- In our experience, if a person is already being fed and content with being fed, then they are unlikely to use an MAS to feed themselves.
- The use of an MAS is most successful when the person living with MND:
  - is motivated to use the equipment
  - is not already being fed by a carer
  - is becoming too tired to finish a meal
  - has a range of movement such that the hand can reach the mouth
  - is supported in a good sitting position
  - has had a recent swallow assessment by a speech and language therapist.

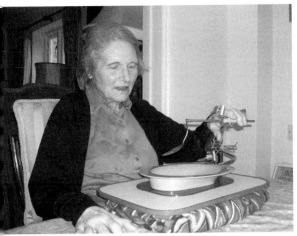

Fig. 11.5 Mobile arm support (reproduced from Talbot K and Marsden R (2008). *Motor Neuron Disease: The Facts,* Oxford University Press, Oxford).

Clothing

Dressing is a daily task that is normally performed with ease and fluency. Therefore, difficulty with dressing is perceived by patients as an early and significant sign of loss of independence. As manual dexterity deteriorates, simple tasks such as doing up buttons can become a very time consuming chore. Alterations can be made to clothing to make dressing and undressing a little easier.

- Shoes should:
  - have good grip
  - have a supportive fit and shape
  - have low heels
  - be fitted with elastic laces
  - be warm in the winter.
- Socks can be put on with a special soft plastic 'sock aid' which rolls into the sock and creates an opening for the foot.
- Underwear:
  - velcro at the sides
  - fine Velcro in gusset area for toilet access.
- Trousers:
  - cord/curtain ring on zip fastener
  - velcro fly
  - elasticized waist
  - one size larger than normally worn
  - braces if belt too difficult to do up.
- Skirts for wheelchair users:
  - open down the back, placed over the knees and tucked in.
- Shirts:
  - velcro placed behind the button.

Beds and chairs

Riser-Recliner chairs

- In order for a person living with MND to be able to relax, comfortable seating is essential. Often family sofas are too low, making it difficult to get up independently.
- Adjustments can be made to existing chairs:
  - blocks to raise the height
  - cushions or pillows to support back, neck, and arms.
- Many people find that Riser-Recliner chairs are the most comfortable. There are many different styles of chair but they tend to have similar functions:
  - electric handset controls
  - a high back for neck and head support
  - reclining back
  - a leg rest
  - well-supported foam seating system
  - tilt forward to aid in standing.
- A single-motor chair tilts the back and legs at the same time, a dual-motor chair allows for more flexibility as the back and legs can be controlled separately.
- These chairs can be bought privately; however, they are also available through the local community occupational therapist or the MND Association.

Beds

Sleep and bed comfort have a major impact on well-being in MND. Nights can be very long if a person is unable to change position, especially if they feel their breathing is compromised. Sleeping habits are formed over a lifetime and are very difficult to change abruptly. People are often very fond of their own bed and reluctant to change.

- Adaptations to an existing bed:
  - blocks under the legs to raise the bed
  - small grab rails to enable turning
  - pillow lifters to enable a raised posture
  - foam wedges, bean bags, or pillows for support
  - mattress overlays for comfort and pressure relief.
- Turning over in bed can be made easier:
  - wear silk night dress or pyjamas
  - use a monkey pole if arm strength is good
  - grab rails on the side of the bed
  - lightweight bed covers, blanket, or duvet.

If these simple adaptations are not sufficient to improve comfort then a special bed may be needed. The impact of moving from a double bed to a single cannot be underestimated and may have a significant impact on a couple's relationship.

Profiling beds

Profiling beds (essentially the same as used in most hospitals) enable changes in position by use of an electronic hand-held control.
The base is divided into separate sections which can be raised or lowered.
A three-section bed allows the back to rise and also the knees to rise to prevent slipping down the bed.
Profiling beds can have as many as five sections of adjustment.
If feeding via a PEG tube and pump overnight then it is recommended that the back of the bed is raised to at least 45° to prevent reflux.
With respiratory compromise, sleeping in an upright position is often the only position of comfort as it allows the chest to expand naturally without the abdominal contents restricting lung capacity.

Mattresses

The correct mattress is essential for comfort and pressure relief.
There are many different manufacturers but essentially three types of mattress:

- memory foam
- alternating air pressure
- water mattress.

Adaptations to the home

Due to the changing nature of disability in motor neuron disease there are many decisions and choices to be made about the home environment. The community OT is the key person in providing assessment and coordinating management of the home environment. They may well also be able to advise on grants that help pay towards the work. However, many community-based therapists only encounter MND patients with a low frequency and will be more used to patients with stable disability (e.g. stroke, trauma). The specialist MND care team has a critical role in educating paramedical colleagues about the progressive nature of the disease in order that they can appropriately prioritize their interventions.

General principles

- It is important not to overwhelm patients by confronting them with all of the disability issues relating to MND at once.
- It is likely that patients with MND will want to put off home adaptations until absolutely necessary, but advance planning is critical to the maintenance of independent living.
- Home adaptations are most likely to be adopted successfully if they are timely and relevant to the current state of disability.
- Informed choice is critical (and should relate to goal planning as outlined previously).
- The rate of disease progression has a major impact on planning adaptations, which have to be completed in a realistic timeframe.
- When considering adaptations to the home it is important to consider
  - How long the work will take?
  - Will it be delivered in a timeframe that provides genuine benefit?
  - Consider the length of time it takes to get finance, planning permission, and engage builders.

Adaptations to the home early in the disease

- Initially, there are simple alterations that can be made without too much disruption, such as:
  - hand rails and handles
  - aids for getting in and out of the bath, e.g. bath boards
  - raised lavatory seats
  - commodes
  - perching stools
  - ramps into and out of the home
  - intercoms.

More significant adaptations

- Using stairs is one of the most significant challenges faced by patients with MND. It may be possible to move the bed downstairs but, if not, consider:
  - stair-lift
  - through-floor lift
  - door widening
  - extension to create a bedroom downstairs.

In the bathroom, access to a shower is very useful. If adaptations are needed consider:

- easy-opening/sliding doors
- non-slip floor
- wheelchair-accessible shower/wet room
- Clos-o-mat™ toilet
- large-handled taps
- lower mirrors.

Environmental control systems

An environmental control system enables a person with significant physical disability to control a range of equipment and appliances using a remote switch and wireless technology. Because of the planning and complexity of such systems at present, they are most likely to be successful in patients with long disease duration.

A system has 3 components:

- **User switch** connected to the control unit. Examples include simple lever, button switch, joy-stick, head switch, suck/puff switch, eye-blink switch.
- **Control unit** which scans though the menu of functions and sends a signal to the selected peripheral device at the activation of the switch. Basic units have just a few functions and more sophisticated units have many hundreds of functions.
- **Peripheral or target devices.** Wide range of appliances broadly categorised into five areas:
  - security, e.g. door entry locks, intercom, alarm or call system
  - access, e.g. door openers and closers
  - communication, e.g. loud-speaker telephone with pre-stored numbers, combined with communication aid
  - equipment operation, e.g. television, radio, lighting, page turner
  - comfort, e.g. electric bed or armchair controls.

Assessment

- Performed by a clinician and/or rehabilitation engineer familiar with motor neuron disease and environmental control systems.
- The choice of switch, control unit, and peripheral devices need to match the user's abilities and needs, which may vary over time.
- Collaboration with the multidisciplinary team over the configuration of the system is important. An environmental control system can be integrated with powered wheelchair controls and some communication aids.

Provision

Services providing environmental control systems vary throughout the UK. Assessment and provision is the responsibility of the local health service. However, additional funding may be available though other government departments such as social services and employment services e.g. Access to work.

Limitations

- An environmental control system should not be provided for 'health' needs as this could put the user at risk in the event of a power cut.
- Environmental control systems can be expensive with costs ranging from around £700 to £5000 and above.

UK suppliers

See Table 11.3.

Table 11.3 UK suppliers of environmental control systems.

Company and address	Examples of controller units
Possum, GEWA and SRS Technology	Primo
	Vivo
Possum Controls Ltd	Freeway and Freeway trolley
8 Farmbrough Close	GEWA Prog
Stocklake Park Industrial Estate	SRS Lite
Aylesbury	SRS Intellec
Buckinghamshire	SRS Mini3
HP20 1DQ	
www.possum.co.uk	
RSL Steeper	Activ500
51 Riverside	
Medway City Estate	
Rochester	
Kent	
ME2 4DP	
www.rslsteeper.com	

Sexual health

- Although MND does not directly cause impairment of sexual function, the impact of the disease can significantly affect physical and sexual relationships.
- Factors influencing sexual relationships:
  - physical disability due to weakness
  - breathlessness due to respiratory muscle involvement
  - cognition
  - emotional responsiveness
  - communication
  - mood
  - fear and anxiety
  - expectations and previous experience
  - changing roles, e.g. from spouse/partner to carer and patient.
- Emotional and physical relationships remain important for people with MND and it is important that health professionals provide opportunities for these personal issues to be discussed. Often, briefly discussing these issues is sufficient to give confidence to the couple to address them in private at home.
- More specific management includes giving simple advice on trying different positions to accommodate weakness and physical disability. More complex psychosexual problems can be referred to a psychosexual practitioner.

Further reading

World Health Organization (2001). ICF: International Classification of Functioning, Disability and Health. WHO.
World Health Organization (1980). ICIDH: International Classification of Impairments, Disability and Handicap. WHO.

End-of-life issues

Mode of death in MND

The overwhelming majority of patients with MND die of their disease rather than incidental causes. Understanding and communicating the way in which people with MND finally die is a matter of critical importance. It is often misrepresented in the non-medical (and unfortunately also in the medical) literature as a sudden and unpleasant death from choking. 'Asphyxiation' is an imprecise term which may be used to mean terminal respiratory failure by physicians but will often be interpreted by patients to mean violent 'suffocation'. Fear of choking to death is an early preoccupation of patients diagnosed with MND. In approximately 500 patients seen in a specialist clinic we have not encountered a patient who had sudden respiratory arrest leading to death during an episode of choking, though the published literature indicates that this may happen very rarely. An accurate picture of the end of life enables the care team to counsel patients effectively, to reduce fear and to facilitate advance planning.

The course of the terminal phase

- The majority of MND patients develop respiratory symptoms in the terminal phase.
- Clinical experience, and limited research, suggests that the mode of death for the vast majority of patients with MND is peaceful, though this is an area where more data are needed.
- The presumed mechanism is progressive hypercapnia with increasing somnolence and ultimately respiratory standstill, often evident as a failure to wake from sleep.
- A minority of patients die suddenly (see Cause of death).
- In studies of the final hours of MND a few per cent of patients are rated by physicians and carers as having 'severe or moderately severe suffering'. Typical symptoms requiring active management include:
  - dyspnoea
  - choking on saliva
  - uncontrollable coughing
  - generalized pain or discomfort.
- Unless active preventive measures are employed (e.g. advance decisions to refuse treatment), there is a small, but very real, risk of patients with MND being subjected to inappropriate resuscitation attempts and admission to intensive care wards.

Cause of death

- It is difficult to gather precise information as even patients who are carefully followed up in specialist clinics will die in a variety of settings and there may be no systematic assessment at the time of death.
- A French study of 302 patients (estimated to be 70% of all deaths expected from ALS in the study population) demonstrated the following causes of death:
  - 77% died of respiratory complications of MND (the majority were recorded as 'terminal respiratory failure', with some cases coded as bronchopneumonia).
  - Pulmonary embolism 2%.
  - Cardiac dysrhythmia 2%.

- Head injury 1.7%.
- Suicide 1.3%.
- <1%: septic shock, MI, haematemesis, and other medical conditions not primarily related to ALS.
- Undetermined 13%.
- The mean disease duration of the patients in this study was 26 months, which might indicate that they did not capture some milder cases.
- Typical ALSFRS scores at death were 15–17, with a range of 9–28 (see Chapter 5), which means that most patients were in a profound state of disability.
- Another French study of 100 patients who underwent autopsy showed a higher rate of pulmonary embolism (6%, mostly spinal-onset patients with lower-limb paralysis) as a likely contributor to the cause of death, and also a significant incidence (10%) of clinically relevant heart failure as a terminal event.

Sudden unexpected death in MND patients

A precise definition of what is sudden and unexpected in a terminal disease is not possible but the term is introduced here to indicate patients who, based on ALSFRS and FVC measures, would normally be expected to live for a period of months, but who die suddenly, usually during sleep.
- This undoubtedly occurs in a minority of patients with MND.
- Causes include:
  - pulmonary embolism (often without clinically obvious leg DVT)
  - cardiac dysrhythmia
  - loss of brainstem respiratory reflex control
  - intentional or inadvertent overdose of medication.
- Even though MND is a terminal illness, it can still come as a great shock to the family of a patient if death supervenes without warning. Identifying those who are at risk of sudden death is not straightforward. However, the following factors are likely to be relevant:
  - rapidly progressing respiratory insufficiency
  - pre-existing cardiac disease
  - recent sub-clinical deep vein thrombosis.

Effect of non-invasive ventilation on end-of-life care

- Although there are methodological issues which make randomized controlled trials in this area difficult, and the primary aim of this therapy is symptom control, there is now limited evidence that NIV prolongs life.
- Much more research is needed to understand how different subgroups of patients respond to NIV.
- For patients with typical ALS, it is likely to prolong the disease for weeks to months.
- In patients in whom respiratory (especially diaphragmatic) weakness is an early and prominent feature there may be a much more pronounced effect on survival.
- Our experience is that the use of NIV does not generally impede end-of-life decision making.
- The use of sedatives, anxiolytics, and narcotics remains the same and the mode of death is not different from MND as a whole.

- In patients on NIV it is doubly important that an advance statement of refusal of treatment has been completed by patients who do not wish to have invasive ventilation.

Mode of death in patients with tracheostomy
- See also Chapter 9.
- 2–3% of patients in case series from specialist clinics have invasive, tracheostomy-assisted ventilation.
- Overall survival after tracheostomy reflects the underlying disease progression and will depend on whether there is selection towards patients with slower progression.
- Death is either due to overwhelming bronchopneumonia or circulatory collapse as a result of the end stage of the neurodegenerative process.
- At the time of death patients are usually in a 'locked-in' state and unable to communicate.
- Terminal weaning under cover of analgesia is one mode of death in invasively ventilated patients.

Place of death in MND
Where people with MND die has consistently proven to be very important to patients and their families. Therefore, it is surprising that there is very little research on the subject, and what does exist demonstrates marked variation across different societies and cultures.
- In observational studies in Europe and North America, the majority of patients die in an institutional setting, either a hospice or an acute hospital.
- For example, in the ALS CARE database, a US multicentre longitudinal observational study in which relatives of patients filled in a questionnaire after the death of the person with MND, 62% of patients died in a 'hospice-supported environment'. Reassuringly, more than 90% of patients had what the relatives judged to be a 'peaceful death'.
- In the UK, where the standard of general practice is high, where there is access to community-based nursing care (District Nurses, Macmillan Nurses etc.), and where Social Services can activate end-of-life care packages, more patients probably die in their own homes. However, data are lacking and there is likely to be considerable variation in practice depending on local resources and care pathways.
- In one combined UK/German study approximately 50% of patients died at home, though the numbers studied were small.

Planning for end-of-life care
- Our experience is that the majority of patients express the wish to die in their own home. The commonest reason why this wish is thwarted is a failure to plan resources effectively, so that home care inevitably breaks down in a crisis.
- The role of the MND care team is to plan ahead to facilitate the wishes of patients dying with MND by:
  - being open and honest about prognosis
  - involving the GP and district nurse
  - establishing good contact with local palliative care teams

- understanding and activating funds available through initiatives such as the 'End-of-life Care Strategy' in the UK, which aims to target resources at those in the terminal phase of their illness (www. endoflifecare.nhs.uk/eolc).
- Hospices, which have long experience of caring for patients dying of cancer, are becoming increasingly orientated towards caring for patients with chronic neurological diseases such as MND. However, MND raises some specific challenges for palliative care specialists:
  - Estimating the prognosis in the terminal phase of MND can be difficult. When resources are limited, hospices may be unwilling to take on the care of MND patients when there is no certainty of death within a defined period.
  - MND treatments such as NIV and PEG, which are intended for symptom control, may be misinterpreted as 'life-prolonging' and lead to confusion about the aims of end-of-life care.
  - Close liaison between the MND care team and palliative care services is required to provide integrated care at the end of life.

Estimating prognosis in the terminal phase

There is a range of reasons why MND specialists are asked to provide a precise estimate of life expectancy:

- Most importantly, many patients value an honest estimate of life expectancy so that they can plan ahead and spread their financial resources accordingly.
- Critical illness and life insurance policies are often triggered when a person is within a specified period from death (often 6 or 12 months).
- End-of-life funding streams (e.g. Continuing Health Care) are activated when a patient is 'rapidly deteriorating'.
- Palliative care services and specifically hospice provision rely on reasonable estimates of life expectancy so that they can use limited resources to good effect.

Evidence base for estimating life expectancy

Numerous studies have established a broadly linear rate of progression in ALS and that a number of measures (ALFRS, FVC) have prognostic value in predicting survival in clinic or trial populations. However, predicting *individual* survival is another matter entirely. The intuition of a clinician experienced in the management of ALS/MND, combined with the measures listed below, may be the best guide to the timing of death:

- The 'referral delay' (i.e. time from symptom onset to diagnosis by an MND neurologist), although a surrogate and retrospective measure, is still the most reliable and independent predictor of overall survival. Shorter delay (<6 months) reflects more aggressive disease.
- Forced vital capacity has been shown to undergo approximately linear decline in ALS. A value below 50% of expected predicts death within 6 months, but with a variation of at least ±3 months. The main problem is that a significant proportion of patients are unable to perform an FVC reliably, and this proportion increases with disease progression.
- Sniff-nasal pressure is not in widespread use but may be technically more reliable in advanced disease, and a value below 40 cmH_2O has a high predictive value for death within 6 months.
- The revised ALSFRS score at initial clinic visit is a reasonable predictor of overall survival. This is likely to be because patients presenting with a lower score have a more rapid disease progression. The slope of the ALSFRS is even more likely to be correlated with survival. A possible advantage of this rating scale is that it does not actually require the presence of the observer and can be administered over the phone or the internet. However, in the terminal phase of the disease it is likely to be less reliable than clinical acumen in predicting survival in individual patients.
- Overall, a skilled clinical neurological specialist in MND can use experience to guide a rough estimate of prognosis which can mostly satisfy the needs outlined above.

- A minority of patients confound medical opinion by dying suddenly or, carrying greater implications for management, continuing past the expected time of their death. This is more likely in patients who have atypical MND with slowly progressive disease, pure lower motor neuron or pure upper motor neuron patterns of involvement, and often younger-onset patients (<50 years).

Advance decisions to refuse treatment

The Mental Capacity Act 2005

The legal framework in the UK for advance directives is the Mental Capacity Act 2005. In the Act, advance directives are referred to as 'Advance Decisions to Refuse Treatment' (ADRT). The Act is underpinned by some key principles:

- A presumption that individuals are capable of making sound decisions about their lives unless it is proved otherwise.
- Individuals must be given every support to enable them to make their own decisions before it is concluded that they are unable to do so.
- Individual decisions must be respected even if these may seem to be different from the norm.
- All decisions made on behalf of a person (without capacity to make their own decisions) must be in their best interests.
- Any intervention on behalf of a person without capacity should be the least restrictive to their basic rights and freedom.
- The Act enables the designation of a decision-maker, called a 'Lasting Power of Attorney' (LPA), who can act on behalf of someone if they lose capacity to make their own decisions. This includes decisions about finances, health care and an advance refusal of treatment. For further information see Mental Capacity Act 2005, Department of Health. Publications and Bulletins or read the Act directly at http://www.opsi.gov.uk/acts/acts2005/20050009.htm

Making an Advance Decision to Refuse Treatment

- An ADRT must be made in writing. A casual remark made in passing does not constitute the basis for an ADRT. If verbal instructions are given and are witnessed, these should be respected and upheld in the normal course of events. However, it is possible that any instructions only given verbally may be ignored in an emergency situation, as refusal to treat may be in conflict with a duty of care.
- There is no required legal wording for completing an ADRT. However it is important that it is clear and succinct. Very wordy documents may be ambiguous and open to misinterpretation at a time when clarity and accuracy are crucial.
- An ADRT does not necessarily have to be drawn up by someone with a legal qualification. Although solicitors are willing to assist people in this regard, our experience is that the resulting document is sometimes vague and 'off-the-peg', and does not address the specific needs of people with MND.
- It is actually very easy for people to make their own ADRT and a number of websites provide templates. However, the assistance of an MND specialist clinic team is advisable as they will have the necessary experience to guide patients through the different decision points in their journey with MND.
- In law, an ADRT is not actually valid if the person to whom it refers retains the capacity to make decisions. ADRTs are therefore only used when the person living with MND is both critically ill and unable to communicate in any way. This is actually a relatively rare situation, but incorrect decisions at this time can have devastating consequences

- It can be very difficult to judge the correct time to raise the subject of advance directives. People with MND should be encouraged to think of an ADRT as an insurance against events that are very unlikely to occur in practice.
- An ADRT should contain some simple information making it clear who 'owns' it, i.e. who is the person to whom it refers, and also who is the principal contact in times of emergency (which may be the same as the next of kin).
- An ADRT technically only covers treatment that the patient does not wish to receive. However, some statements which are more specific to MND may be included, such as:
  - The preferred place of care in the terminal phase and the circumstances under which hospital admission is acceptable.
  - What to do in the event of a chest infection. If the infection is not controlled by oral antibiotics should treatment continue in hospital with intravenous therapy?
  - In the situation where someone is at the end of life but unconscious there may be concern about discomfort from dehydration. In general this is not an issue in MND and should not be the prime reason for hospital or hospice admission. It is good practice to record if there is a strong feeling about hydration.
  - Morphine and related drugs are commonly used for symptom control in terminal care in MND but can suppress respiratory drive. It is important to record that possible negative effects of morphine are accepted as a justified price to pay for good symptom relief.
  - What to do in the event of a cardiorespiratory arrest. It is critical that this is documented and easily accessible to emergency medical and paramedical personnel in order to avoid accidental resuscitation. A statement in an ADRT indicating that someone wishes to have all care to support their well-being and comfort but not to have their life artificially prolonged by invasive (i.e. tracheostomy-assisted) ventilation is an important way of avoiding this outcome.

An ADRT should be signed and dated by the person to whom it refers and also by a witness. The number of copies that have been made and their location should be documented. In the event that the ADRT is changed or rewritten, the first version should be destroyed.
We generally advise the following:

- The Lions Club (www.lions.org.uk/miab.htm) can provide a 'message in a bottle'. The ADRT is placed in the bottle which is then kept in the refrigerator. A sticker with a green cross placed on the front and back doors alerts any emergency services that there is important medical information in the fridge, chosen because it is normally in the kitchen and easy to locate. Some GP practices routinely use this scheme, but they can also be obtained directly from the Lions Club. Some people decide to keep one copy on their person or in a hand bag, give one copy to the next of kin, and one copy is retained by the GP.

- In some areas the local ambulance control will be happy to indicate the fact that someone has an ADRT on their database. Thus if an ambulance is ever called they will be alerted to the fact that someone in the household has an ADRT.
- In the UK a copy of an ADRT can also be sent to NHS Direct which now has a national database and a system for flagging up special instructions.

Exit strategies

The nature of motor neuron disease, with relentless progression, lack of effective treatment, and the inevitability of death, have placed it at the centre of the debate about voluntary euthanasia and physician-assisted suicide. In many ways this has had unfortunate consequences for sufferers of the disease, their carers, and health-care professionals, whose voices often seem lost within this debate. The worst aspects of MND (loss of control, paralysis, dependence, loss of communication) and things that either happen rarely, or not at all, are brought to prominence by advocates of assisted suicide or by the broadcast and print media. It is common in this context to read of MND causing death through suffocation or choking.

Wishes and intentions of patients with respect to hastened death

- Precise data is lacking, but it is reasonable to assume that many patients are reticent about discussing this with members of the care team, and that the incidence is higher than evident from clinical practice.
- In a study of ALS patients in Oregon, 56% responded affirmatively to the statement 'under some circumstances I would consider taking a prescription for a medicine whose sole purpose was to end my life'.
- Positive responders were more likely to be male, educated, non-religious, and score highly on measures of hopelessness (but not depression).
- The majority considered that they would gain comfort from knowing that such an option was available without actually acting on it, suggesting that a sense of empowerment and control is an important factor.
- There are no exact figures in the UK for those who have shortened their own lives, bearing in mind that physician-assisted suicide and euthanasia are both illegal. In our own clinical practice we estimate the number to be 2–3% of patients with typical ALS.

Physician-assisted suicide

There are a number of locations in which physician-assisted suicide (defined as voluntarily taking a medication at a lethal dose, prescribed by a physician, with the express intention of ending one's life) is practiced within a legal framework:

- Netherlands, Belgium, Oregon (USA)
- The law is permissive, in the sense of not prosecuting physicians, in Switzerland.

Brain donation and banking

Neuropathology provides fundamental insights which underpin our current understanding of MND and other neurodegenerative disorders, as well as insights into the marked clinical heterogeneity in MND. The identification of ubiquitinated inclusions, and latterly TDP-43 as a major protein constituent, demonstrate the vital importance of access to autopsy material from MND patients. Many patients are highly motivated to leave a 'legacy' to researchers in the form of a gift of their brain and spinal cord. Clinicians should strive to do everything possible to honour this wish.

- Raising the subject of brain donation is potentially very awkward and careful judgment is needed. It is rarely, if ever, appropriate at the time of diagnosis.
- The provision of written material in the form of research 'newsletters' or on a clinic website are examples of ways in which interested patients can be informed without risking offending the sensibilities of patients who do not wish to consider this option.
- Obtaining pre-mortem consent is of uncertain legal validity but has the very important purpose of making the wishes of the potential donor clear to their families and GP, which greatly facilitates the logistics of donation after death.
- A post-mortem consent form must be completed by the next of kin after death.
- In counseling next of kin the following should be made clear:
  - Once the patient has died the arrangements for storage of the body by funeral directors should proceed as normal.
  - The neuropathology department which issued the original consent should be contacted in office hours and they will generally liaise with the funeral director.
  - There will be no delay in funeral arrangements.
  - If the brain and spinal cord only are removed, this will be achieved without any change in the external appearance of the body.
  - Results from neuropathological analysis will take 2–3 months.
  - Feedback will always be given to the family unless directed otherwise.
- A list of UK departments willing to facilitate the collection autopsy material from patients with MND can be found on the MND Association website at: www.mndassociation.org/search_clicks.rm?id=8 1&destinationtype=2&instanceid=138614

Further reading

Albert SM, Rabkin JG, Del Bene ML *et al.* (2005). Wish to die in end-stages of ALS. *Neurology,* 65, 68–74.

Ganzini I, Johnston WS, McFarland BH, Tolle SW, Lee MA. (1998). Attitudes of patients with ALS and their caregivers toward assisted suicide. *N Engl J Med,* 339, 967–973.

Gil J, Funalot B, Verschueren A *et al.* (2008). Causes of death amongst French patients with amyotrophic lateral sclerosis: a prospective study. *Eur J Neurol,* 15, 1245–51.

Veldinik JH, Wokke JH, van der Wal G, Vianney de Jong JM, van den Berg LH (2002). Euthanasia and physician-assisted suicide among patients with ALS in the Netherlands. *N Engl J Med,* 346, 1638–1644.

Carers and families

Carer burden

The effects of a disease like MND inevitably extend beyond the patient and have an enormous impact on family, friends, and colleagues. Those living with someone with MND may only watch as day by day changes occur which they are powerless to stop. Partners and friends may find themselves in the unexpected position of caring for their loved one.

- A carer can be defined as someone who is caring for a partner, friend, or child but does not have a paid contract of work. This care normally takes place in the dependant's own home.
- The 2001 UK Census identified that there were 5.2 million carers living in England and Wales. This equates to 1 in 10 of the population. One million of these carers provide more than 50 hours care per week.
- Thus carers provide the vast majority of care for people in this country.
- Studies have shown:
  - Carers are likely to have emotional and mental health issues, particularly in complaining of fatigue and physical problems like back ache.
  - If carers do not seek help and support it is possible for them to become isolated, unable to leave the house due to their caring responsibilities.

Rights of carers

- In 2000 the Carers and Disabled Children Act allowed carers who were aged 16 or over and provided a regular and substantial amount of care for someone aged 18 or over to have the right to a needs assessment which is carried out by Social Services.
- In 2004 the Carers Equal Opportunities Act increased the rights of carers. If a carer wishes to undertake study or leisure activity this should be taken into account. The aim is to encourage Carers to have time to pursue their own interests.

Respite care

Carers must consider if the care they are providing is sustainable in the long term. They should be reassured that it is not a sign of weakness or failure to accept help and support. The type and amount of help available will depend on resources in the local area, and the wish to supplement this using individual financial reserves.

- Examples of different types of care that may be available:
  - Care given in suitable accommodation for a fixed period of time, e.g. a local community hospital, disability centre, hospice, or even hotel.
  - Domiciliary care by paid care staff from an agency assisting with the care needs either at set times during the day or for a continuous block of time. The structure of this care should reflect the normal carer's needs as well as those of the person living with MND.
  - Day care delivered out of the home environment, returning home in the afternoon. This may take place once or twice a week. Day care often provides ongoing assessment for the person attending as well as respite for their carer.
- In addition to the limitations imposed by constraints on resources, there are a number of barriers to acceptance of help with care:
  - The knowledge that the remaining time that can be spent with a person with a terminal illness is necessarily limited can induce a sense of guilt about leaving them, even for short periods.
  - Dependence of the person being cared for, who may not easily accept someone else unfamiliar with their precise needs.
  - Loss of privacy.
- By slowly introducing 'outside helpers' and enabling them to get to know the person living with MND the circle of trust may gradually grow to incorporate other people as well as the main carer.
- Sharing some of the burden of care may make the situation more sustainable and prevent a crisis.

Sources of support for carers

- The MND Association
  - The website offers a great deal of specific information for carers (www.mndassociation.org).
  - MND Connect (08457 626262) is a helpline.
  - Most areas have a local branch of the MND Association which can give individual support to both the person living with MND and their partner, family, and friends.
  - Regional Care Development Advisors and Association Visitors offer ongoing advice and support to people living with MND, their family, friends, and health care professionals. To find a local one call 08457 626262.
- Health and Social Care: can organize an initial visit and carry out a Carers Assessment.
- Carers UK (www.carersuk.org) has the power to lobby on behalf of carers; it also has a forum for carers to communicate online.
- The Carers Centre (www.thecarerscentre.org) is a national network which gives carers support and information, including practical assistance in filling out forms, applying for grant applications, etc.

Young families affected by MND

- Living with MND is hard enough. Patients with young families have the added anguish of:
  - caring for their children whilst they are disabled
  - extra fatigue, especially when caring for small children
  - dealing with their own grief and sense of bereavement for the loss of seeing their children grow up
  - worrying about who will care for their children in the long term.
- Parents naturally want to protect their child from what is happening to themselves. However, children are extremely sensitive to change and good at detecting when things are not right. Therefore, honesty and openness, at a level suitable to the child's age and understanding, is the best policy.
- Personal contact with the child's school teachers may help them interpret changes in behaviour and academic performance at school.
- Parents should be gently encouraged to think about ways in which they can leave a legacy for children (see www.winstonswish.org.uk):
  - writing letters to the child
  - making a diary
  - making a video tape/DVD
  - leaving personal gifts
  - a 'memory box' which my contain a favourite perfume, photographs, written memories
  - letters for the future.
- There is a great deal of support available to families:
  - www.SeeSaw.org helps children and their families both before and after a major bereavement, helping them to move forward.
  - www.winstonswish.org.uk/ helps children to rebuild their lives after the death of a parent or sibling.
  - www.childhoodbereavementnetwork.org.uk The services in this directory can be contacted for information, guidance, and support by anyone caring for or working with a bereaved child or young person in the UK.
  - www.childbeareavement.org.uk This helps families understand the grieving process. It gives advice on how a school can help and provides guidance on developing a policy and training courses for all professionals.
  - www.crusebereavementcare.org.uk/ Cruse is the national bereavement charity. It provides advice on helping young people.

Other motor neuron disorders

Classification of motor neuron disorders

The World Federation of Neurology Classification of Neurological Disease lists over 100 disorders which involve motor neurons. In the absence of a clear understanding of aetiology in all cases, classification is based on a number of axes including clinical features (UMN vs LMN) and inheritance pattern if relevant. For the reasons mentioned in Chapter 6 the exact distinction between familial and sporadic ALS is blurred by the existence of patients with apparent sporadic ALS but mutations in genes such as SOD1, TDP-43, FUS, and angiogenin. Similarly there are patients with the phenotype of HSP or SMA who do not have a family history and may be examples of genuinely sporadic analogues of these normally genetically determined conditions. The classification below is a brief and simplified overview and does not include every known motor neuron disorder or complex CNS disorder where motor neuron involvement is a minor feature:

- Genetic:
  - Pure UMN (hereditary spastic paraparesis):
    - More than 30 genetic variants.
    - Classified as pure or complex (other neurological features).
  - Pure LMN (spinal muscular atrophy/hereditary motor neuropathy):
    - Recessive.
    - Dominant.
    - X-linked (SBMA).
  - Mixed UMN/LMN (familial ALS):
    - ALS1–11.
  - ALS-FTD (ALS with frontotemporal dementia).
- Sporadic degenerative:
  - Pure UMN (primary lateral sclerosis).
  - Pure lower motor neuron (progressive muscular atrophy).
  - Mixed UMN/LMN (amyotrophic lateral sclerosis) +/- frontotemporal dementia.
  - Western Pacific ALS.
  - Segmental (monomelic amyotrophy).
- Inflammatory:
  - Pure motor CIDP.
  - Multifocal motor neuropathy with conduction block.
- Infective:
  - Poliomyelitis.
  - Other viruses: Japanese B encephalitis, West Nile virus.
  - HIV disease with motor neuron involvement.
- Toxic/nutritional:
  - Konzo.
  - Lathyrism.
  - Mercury poisoning.
- Paraneoplastic:
  - Motor neuronopathy in non-Hodgkin's lymphoma.
  - PLS-like syndrome in breast cancer.

Kennedy's disease

- X-linked.
- Incidence 1 in 40,000.
- Translated CAG expansion in the first exon of the androgen receptor (AR) gene.
- Results in the expression of a protein with an expanded polyglutamine (polyGln) sequence in its N-terminal.
- Gain of function mutation due to acquired cellular toxicity of polyglutamine protein (complete loss of AR in testicular feminization syndrome does not lead to motor neuron degeneration).
- Significant effect in males only.
- Length of CAG expansion correlates with age of onset but apparently not rate of disease progression.
- Rare manifesting carrier females have been described with cramps (50% of female carriers have mild chronic denervation on EMG).
- Median onset 50 years (range 30–70).
- Characteristic clinical features makes confusion with ALS unlikely:
  - postural tremor
  - cramps and fasciculations (esp. perioral fasciculations)
  - tongue wasting but very little evidence of weakness
  - symmetrical proximal > distal weakness and wasting (LL>UL)
  - areflexia
  - signs of partial androgen insensitivity (gynaecomastia present in 50%, reduced fertility).
- Slow progression (Japanese study of 223 patients):
  - average age of onset of tremor 33 years
  - lower limb weakness, 44 years
  - dysathria, 49 years
  - dysphagia, 54 years
  - use of a stick by 59 years
  - wheelchair by 65 years
  - very slow progression with little effect on lifespan
  - 30% lose ambulation by 65.
- Diagnosis:
  - Genetic test routinely available.
  - PCR of expanded region of AR.
  - Range of expansions: normal 9–36, affected 40–62 CAG repeats.
  - CPK typically elevated 3–4 fold.
  - NCS/EMG: consistent but mild sensory neuropathy.
- Management of disability, gait disturbance, and respiratory function.
- Experimental treatment:
  - Androgen receptor blockade.
  - Rationale: motor neuron degeneration thought to be due to excess AR stimulation in men driven by elevated testosterone.

Post-polio syndrome

- Definition (Halstead criteria, 1991):
  - history of poliomyelitis with partial or complete functional recovery
  - stable function for >15 years
  - onset of two or more of: functional loss, extensive fatigue, muscle pain, new weakness, new muscle atrophy, cold intolerance
  - no other medical explanation (so in practice a diagnosis of exclusion).
- Incidence: varies widely (15–80% of all people with previous polio) according to how criteria are applied.
- There is lack of agreement on whether the appearance of new weakness and wasting is necessary to diagnose PPS.
- Role of neurophysiology:
  - demonstration of lower motor neuron degeneration and its extent
  - exclusion of other causes of weakness such as entrapment.
- Slowly progressive.
- Complex and uncertain aetiology:
  - no evidence of reactivation of latent poliovirus
  - possible contribution of failure of compensation for age-related motor unit loss on the background of depleted reserve
  - co-morbidities (e.g. osteoarthritis) are an important determinant of disability.
- Therapy:
  - Pyridostigmine, prednisolone (80 mg/day), and amantidine have all been used for weakness and fatigue, but in each case there is trial evidence of no benefit.
  - Concerns that overuse of muscles lead to accelerated weakness have not been substantiated by evidence. Patients who report regular physical activity have reduced levels of disability by improving general fitness and well-being. The benefit of graded and supervised exercise programs is supported by short-term, small-scale studies, but more evidence over the long term is required.
  - Exercise in a warm swimming pool seems to be helpful.
- Respiratory function is normal in most patients, but those who were ventilated in acute illness and those with significant chest deformity are at risk of nocturnal hypoventilation and sleep-disordered breathing.
- General advice such as weight loss, provision of aids such as splints, psychological support.

Autosomal recessive spinal muscular atrophy

- Clinically divided into 4 types by maximum motor milestones:
  - Type I: infantile onset ('floppy baby'), survival 0–18 months without assisted ventilation. Poor head control and weak cough. Intercostal weakness with diaphragmatic sparing leads to characteristic paradoxical breathing with abdominal expansion.
  - Type II: can sit but never walk. Fine finger tremor. Prognosis depends on degree of respiratory weakness. Kyphoscoliosis requires corrective spinal bracing and surgery.
  - Type III: can stand unaided. Normal lifespan. 40% lose ambulation by age 50.
  - Type IV: adult onset (genetically heterogeneous).
- Clinical features:
  - Proximal wasting and weakness.
  - Tongue fasciculation in Type I.
  - Sparing of facial muscles until late in disease.
  - Legs affected more than arms in milder forms.
  - After initial onset progression is slow.
  - Disability in childhood-onset forms in part related to growth of axial skeleton outstripping neuromuscular territory.
- Molecular basis:
  - Autosomal recessive: patients are compound heterozygotes for deletions and gene conversion events between SMN1 and copy gene SMN2. Copy number of SMN2 determines overall severity.
  - Inactivating mutations in the SMN gene reduce level of SMN protein to 15–20% of normal.
  - Diagnosis is by PCR to identify deletions of SMN1 (<3% of patients carry point mutations on one chromosome).
- Cellular basis:
  - A neurodegenerative disease, a neurodevelopmental disease, or both?
  - SMN functions in all cells as a co-factor in the biogenesis of small ribonucleoprotein (snRNP) necessary for efficient splicing.
  - Putative distinct function in axons associated with transport and translational control of specific mRNAs down axon to neuromuscular junction.
- Management limited to experimental treatments:
  - Aimed at increasing SMN protein levels by altering epigenetic expression from SMN2 locus.
  - Histone deacetylase inhibitors in clinical trial.
  - Albuterol (sympathomimetic) anecdotally slightly improves function.

Miscellaneous lower motor neuron syndromes

- Many different conditions characterised by slowly progressive neurogenic weakness and wasting are described.
- Confusion is caused by a lack of consistency in the use of the term 'spinal muscular atrophy':
  - 'Progressive SMA' is used by some neurologists as a synonym for the PMA form of motor neuron disease, which is also known simply as 'lower motor neuron disease'. Conceptually, these patients belong in the spectrum of ALS-like MND on the grounds of pace of change and common findings at autopsy.
  - Neurophysiologists are prone to apply the term to patients with chronic 'denervation and re-innervation'.
- Slowly progressive distal wasting and weakness is often inherited in an autosomal dominant pattern:
  - The terms 'Hereditary Motor Neuropathy' and 'distal SMA' are essentially synonyms for the same condition.
  - This resembles a pure motor axonal form of Charcot-Marie-Tooth disease. Some of these patients have mild sensory loss and they are then referred to as CMT2.
  - A common clinical pattern is progressive peroneal muscular atrophy with pes cavus and mild or late involvement of the hands. A small proportion of these cases have mutations in the small heat shock protein genes hsp22 or hsp27.
  - Mutations in the gene for glycyl t-RNA synthetase (GARS) cause a form of dominant motor neuropathy (HMN7 of dSMA Type V) characterised by early hand involvement.
  - Some families with SPG17 (Silver syndrome) contain individuals with isolated distal weakness and wasting of the hands.
- There are rare families with dominant inheritance of a condition that resembles autosomal recessive proximal SMA. The gene has not been identified. The main differential is limb-girdle muscular dystrophy.
- The term 'asymmetrical SMA' is a label applied to rare patients (often young men) who have an extended form of segmental lower motor neuron degeneration, the aetiology of which is likely to be heterogeneous and at present remains obscure. It is very slowly progressive.

Monomelic amyotrophy

- Also known as Hirayama's disease or segmental SMA.
- Weakness and wasting largely confined to one limb, usually upper.
- Heterogeneous condition.
- In young males from Japan or India/Pakistan there is a distinct syndrome:
  - Onset late teens or early 20s.
  - C6–8 segments affected.
  - Insidious onset over a few months.
  - Arrests or only slowly progressive.
  - Never familial, despite strong ethnic predisposition.
  - Aetiology obscure: reports of compression from dural sac on MRI but not in all cases. Autopsy shows focal loss of ventral horn motor neurons ('poliodystrophy').
  - 20–30% have mild contralateral changes.
  - Lower limb monomelic atrophy is described but does not show the same geographical distribution.
- The distinction from ALS, which often presents with involvement in the upper limb, is based mainly on the pattern of progression:
  - There is usually some evidence on first presentation of ALS of upper motor neuron signs and sub-clinical involvement outside of the affected limb.
  - Clear progression to another limb within 3–6 months in ALS.
  - Prominent fasciculation in ALS.
- Differential diagnosis of weakness and wasting in one upper limb:
  - brachial neuritis
  - polyradiculopathy
  - multifocal motor neuropathy with conduction block
  - inclusion body myositis, though this is usually bilateral but asymmetrical.
- There remain other patients who do not fit into these categories. Occasional patients report trauma as a remote or recent background event, but a causal relationship is uncertain.
- Hopkin's syndrome is a very rare condition, which usually presents in childhood, and consists of weakness and wasting of one arm which occurs some weeks after an acute episode of asthma treated with steroids.

Hereditary spastic paraparesis

- Progressive spastic paraparesis implies a degenerative process involving the long axons of the corticospinal tract.
- The core clinical syndrome consists of:
  - Increased tone in the lower limbs leading to a narrow-based 'spastic gait', associated with brisk reflexes, clonus, and extensor plantar responses.
  - Weakness is not a prominent feature.
  - Mild and often sub-clinical sensory loss at ankles.
- The differential diagnosis includes:
  - compressive lesions of the spinal cord
  - hereditary spastic paraparesis
  - B12 deficiency (sub-acute combined degeneration of the cord)
  - primary progressive multiple sclerosis
  - copper deficiency myelopathy
  - adrenomyeloneuropathy
  - tropical spastic paraparesis.
- Hereditary spastic paraparesis (HSP) is conventionally divided into:
  - Pure HSP, in which there is no associated involvement of other neurological systems. This is more likely to be dominantly inherited and onset varies from childhood to middle age.
  - Complicated HSP, in which a variety of other neurological systems are affected, leading to ataxia, optic atrophy, mental retardation, deafness, epilepsy, peripheral neuropathy, etc. These conditions are more likely to be recessive or X linked and early in onset.
- More than 40 different genetic loci, many very rare (single families).
- Autosomal recessive forms of HSP:
  - SPG7, Paraplegin (pure)
  - SPG11, Spatacsin (associated with thin corpus callosum).
- X-linked forms of HSP:
  - SPG2, PLP gene, Pelizaeus-Merzbacher
  - adrenomyeloneuropathy (progressive myelopathy due to mutations in the ALD gene, which in males more commonly causes infantile adrenoleucodystrophy. 40% of female carriers are affected by progressive spastic paraparesis beginning in middle life; diagnosis by elevation of very long chain fatty acid levels)
- Autosomal dominant forms of HSP:
  - SPG4, Spastin (40% of pure HSP); Atlastin (10%)
  - SPG17, Silver Syndrome (+distal wasting of hands and pes cavus), mutations in BSCL2.
- Function of mutated proteins suggests that axonal transport, protein chaperones, and mitochondrial function are important pathways.
- Management:
  - Adult onset forms are generally slowly progressive over decades.
  - Gait disturbance dominated by spasticity, weakness is distal and mild.
  - Mild bladder urgency responds to anti-cholinergics.
  - Anti-spasticity agents generally limited by side effects and lack of efficacy.

Further reading

Atsuta N, Watanabe H, Ito M, *et al.* (2006). Natural history of spinal and bulbar muscular atrophy (SBMA): a study of 223 Japanese patients. *Brain*, 29, 1446–55.

Farbu E, Gilhus NE, Barnes MP, *et al.* (2006). EFNS guideline on diagnosis and management of post-polio syndrome. Report of an EFNS task force. *Eur J Neurol*, 13, 795–801.

Wang CH, Finkel RS, Bertini ES, *et al.* (2007). Consensus Statement for Standard of Care in Spinal Muscular Atrophy. *J Child Neurol*, 22, 1027–49.

Useful internet-based sources of information

There are many sources of information about MND and related disorders available to patients via the internet. We have only included below those sites with which we are familiar and for which the web address is likely to remain constant over time. The internet is a great force for freedom of information but clearly sites designed for patients will be most useful if there is guidance from the MND team. Most of the sites below will contain information of value to both professionals and patients.

Useful websites for professionals

- ALSOD: http://alsod.iop.kcl.ac.uk/Als/index.aspx
  - An online database of genetic mutations in ALS.
- ALS Therapy Development Institute: www.als.net
  - A charitably funded foundation dedicated to developing new drug treatments for ALS.
- Washington University Neuromuscular Disease Center: http://neuromuscular.wustl.edu
  - A superb resource for neurologists with an interest in neuromuscular disease.
- GeneTests: www.geneclinics.org
  - Expert reviews on genetic conditions.
- TREAT-NMD: www.treat-nmd.eu/home.php
  - A research network for clinical trials in neuromuscular diseases.

ALS Patient support groups

- Motor Neuron Disease Association (UK): www.mndassociation.org
  - Provides a wide range of general information about MND. Information specific to the UK, such as the location of MNDA-funded care centres is also included.
  - MND Association Help Line: 08457 626262.
- ALS Association (USA): www.alsa.org
  - This is a very comprehensive site which has up to date information about research as well as factual information about ALS.
- Synapse (USA): www.synapsepls.org
  - A website specifically devoted to primary lateral sclerosis.
- The International Alliance of ALS/MND Associations: www. alsmndalliance.org
  - This provides international information which can link anyone living with MND to the clinics and organizations relevant to their locality.

Patient support groups for other motor neuron diseases

- Jennifer Trust for Spinal Muscular Atrophy (UK): www.jtsma.org.uk
- SMA Trust (UK): www.smatrust.org
- Families of SMA (USA): www.fsma.org
- SMA Foundation (USA): www.smafoundation.org
- Kennedy's Disease Association (USA): www.kennedysdisease.org
- UK HSP Support Group: www.hspgroup.org
- Spastic Paraplegia Foundation (USA): www.sp-foundation.org

Driving

- Government advice about driving (UK) including Blue Badge scheme: www.direct.gov.uk/en/DisabledPeople/MotoringAndTransport
- DVLA medical rules: www.dvla.gov.uk/medical.aspx

Sources of practical information for patients

- RADAR: www.radar.org.uk
  - A national network of disability campaigning groups.
- The Neurological Alliance: www.neural.org.uk
  - Campaigning for people with neurological disease.
- Health Talk (formerly DIPex) (UK): www.healthtalkonline.org
  - A site devoted to personal experiences of health and illness. People can watch, listen to, or read interviews with people suffering from various diseases including MND and find reliable information on treatment choices and where to find support.
- Travel advice:
  - www.dialuk.info and www.radar.org.uk are useful resources about travel for people with disabilities.
  - www.doctorbabel.com offers a service where medical details can be translated into any of the common languages.
  - Travel insurance: the MNDA website contains up-to-date information about companies which are happy to insure people with MND.
- Benefits:
  - The benefits enquiry line 0800 882200 is a helpline to explain entitlement to benefits and ensure appropriate forms are sent out.
- Citizens Advice Bureau: www.citizensadvice.org.uk
  - The national office is 0207 833 2181 and provides details of local offices.
  - Address:
    Citizens Advice
    Myddelton House, 115–123 Pentonville Road,
    London N1 9LZ
- DIAL UK: www.dialuk.info
  - A national advice line with 130 local branches to provide local disability information, advice, and support.
  - Telephone: 01302 310 123.
  - Address:
    St Catherine's
    Tickhill Road
    Doncaster
    South Yorkshire
    DN4 8QN

Index